MCQ

EXAMINATIONS IN PSYCHIATRY

AUP titles of related interest

MODELS FOR PSYCHOTHERAPY, A PRIMER
J D Haldane, D A Alexander, L G Walker

A CELEBRATION OF MARRIAGE?
Scotland 1931–81: implications for marital counselling and therapy
J D Haldane

THE MALCOLM MILLAR LECTURES

THE PSYCHODYNAMIC IMAGE OF MAN
a philosophy for the caring professions
J D Sutherland

CONSULTATIVE WORK WITH COMMUNITIES AND ORGANISATIONS
towards a psychodynamic image of man
Harold Bridger

THERAPY AND CARE
psychodynamic and theological images of man
G R Dunstan

PSYCHOTHERAPY AND THE PRACTICE OF CHILD PSYCHIATRY
Fred H Stone

CONFLICT AND STRESS
the significant role of community psychotherapy
Francis A Macnab

RESEARCH AND THE PRACTICE OF PSYCHOTHERAPY
M G Gelder

MCQ

EXAMINATIONS IN PSYCHIATRY

John M Eagles
David A Alexander

ABERDEEN UNIVERSITY PRESS

First published 1986
Aberdeen University Press
A member of the Pergamon Group

© John M Eagles and David A Alexander 1986

British Library Cataloguing in Publication Data

Eagles, John M
    MCQ examinations in psychiatry
    1. Psychiatry—Problems, exercises, etc.
    I. Title II. Alexander, D A
    616.89'0076   RC457

    ISBN 0 08 032472 X

Printed in Great Britain
The University Press
Aberdeen

CONTENTS

ACKNOWLEDGEMENTS

We wish to thank Dr D. P. K. Brown for his comments on and contributions to the questions on mental handicap. We are also grateful to Professor G. W. Ashcroft, Dr J. A. O. Besson, Dr K. P. Ebmeier, Dr J. D. Hendry and Dr L. G. Walker for their useful comments and advice. To our local psychiatric trainees we are also indebted for giving us their suggestions and opinions on our questions from the consumers' point of view. Finally, we appreciate the patient co-operation of Miss Sybil McLeod in the typing of the manuscript.

PREFACE

This book is principally focused on the requirements of trainees in psychiatry who are preparing for the MRC Psych. Examination, but it should also constitute a useful form of "revision" for post-graduates both in psychiatry and in other disciplines. For the psychiatric trainee, the book is intended to provide a means both of revising knowledge and of gaining expertise in completing Multiple Choice Questionnaire Examinations. While the place of the MCQ in medical examinations has been questioned (e.g. Pickering, 1979), it currently constitutes the principal method for testing the "factual" knowledge of post-graduates in psychiatric training.

MCQs do test factual knowledge—and candidates with insufficient knowledge will fail—but success in MCQs also requires an appropriate examination technique. General aspects of this technique are described by Anderson (1982). Probably the most vexatious component of a good MCQ technique is knowing "when to guess and when not to guess". That this factor can have considerable bearing on an examinee's scores has been shown by Sanderson (1973) and by Harden et al (1976). With this in mind, each question in the book is followed by three columns headed Certain ("Ctn"), Doubtful ("Dbt") and Guess ("Gu"). Examinees vary with regard to how accurately and how readily they "guess", and this system will allow you to reach a clearer view of the "level of certainty" at which you should opt for a "True" or a "False" rather than a "Don't Know".

The composition of our papers is designed to reflect that of the Royal College of Psychiatrists' "sample" paper, as well as that of recent Membership examinations. The degree of difficulty of the questions, in our view, slightly exceeds that of the Membership examination. To avoid lulling candidates into a false sense of security by setting questions at too simple a level, we considered that the educational contribution of the book was best served by erring on the side of stretching the readers.

Answers and explanations follow the question papers. Space does not permit a lengthy exposition on each question and, thus, references are provided for readers who wish to research the topic more fully. These references also back our assertions as to the "accuracy" of the answers we have provided. We have attempted to design questions where the facts are not in dispute. However, in psychiatry, facts are not immutable, and a few of our "facts" may have even been disproved by the time this book is published!

John M Eagles
David A Alexander
April, 1986

PAPER 1

	Ctn	Dbt	Gu

1.1 School refusers:

(a) tend to be of below average IQ.

(b) often have depressed mothers.

(c) tend to be unduly reliant on their
mothers.

(d) are most commonly 5 to 7 years old.

(e) rarely show persisting problems
after regular school attendance
is achieved.

1.2 Child abuse is:

(a) less likely among very young parents.

(b) usually reported immediately by the
abusing parents to avoid detection.

(c) less likely towards premature babies.

(d) associated with high levels of
verbal interaction between the
child and the abusing mother.

(e) more likely among unemployed
parents.

	Ctn	Dbt	Gu

1.3 Children who set fires:

(a) are usually boys.

(b) usually do so alone.

(c) usually commit other offences as well.

(d) tend to be from strict middle-class homes.

(e) are usually older than other conduct disordered children.

1.4 The following are typical of Gilles de la Tourette's syndrome.

(a) Epileptiform seizures.

(b) Multiple tics.

(c) Coprolalia.

(d) Onset between age 20 and 50 years.

(e) Auditory hallucinations.

1.5 **The following statements about**
delinquency are correct.

(a) Teachers' ratings of the child's
behaviour at primary school are not
predictive of delinquent behaviour
in adolescence.

                                                        — — —

(b) The friends and relatives of delinquents
have a high incidence of criminality.

    — — —

(c) The majority of delinquents do not
go on to a life of adult crime.

    — — —

(d) Delinquents differ significantly
from non-delinquents on various
psychophysiological measures.

    — — —

(e) Delinquents differ significantly
from non-delinquents in their
incidence of EEG abnormalities.

    — — —

1.6 **In children the following statements**
apply to nocturnal enuresis.

(a) It is commoner in children of lower
social class.

    — — —

(b) There is an increased risk if one of
the child's parents was similarly
affected.

    — — —

(c) Anxiety-provoking events in early
childhood increase the likelihood
of its occurrence.

    — — —

(d) Its occurrence usually indicates
that a child is emotionally
disturbed.

    — — —

(e) There is a significant association
with urinary tract infection.

    — — —

4

1.7 Cri du chat syndrome is associated with:

(a) low set ears.

(b) a characteristic mewing cry.

(c) a high morbidity rate in infancy.

(d) macrocephaly.

(e) webbing of the neck.

1.8 The following statements about phenylketonuria (PKU) are correct.

(a) It is transmitted as a recessive autosomal trait.

(b) The majority of patients with PKU have only mild intellectual handicap.

(c) PKU children are rarely hyperactive.

(d) Early diagnosis is important for effective treatment.

(e) The Guthrie test is a screening method for PKU.

1.9 The following are recognised clinical features of Down's syndrome.

(a) Stereotypies.

(b) Clinodactyly.

(c) Brachycephaly.

(d) Brushfield spots.

(e) Echolalia.

	Ctn	Dbt	Gu

1.10 The following are autosomal dominant disorders.

(a) Tuberous sclerosis (epiloia).

(b) Neurofibromatosis (von Recklinghausen's disease).

(c) Wilson's disease.

(d) Lesch - Nyhan syndrome.

(e) Marfan's syndrome.

1.11 Systematic desensitization:

(a) derives from the work of Wolpe.

(b) is the same as response prevention.

(c) should not be used with hypnosis.

(d) involves the construction of a hierarchy of anxiety-provoking stimuli.

(e) substitutes constructive responses for maladaptive ones.

1.12 The following have a specific relevance to family therapy.

(a) Multiple impact therapy.

(b) The "empty nest syndrome".

(c) Sculpting.

(d) Collective unconscious.

(e) Circular reaction.

**1.13   In general, the behavioural approach
to treatment:**

(a)   emphasizes the value of insight by the
patient.

                                              ___   ___   ___

(b)   regards overt behaviour change as the
major criterion in evaluating treatment
outcome.

                                              ___   ___   ___

(c)   specifies treatment procedures in
objective and operational terms.

                                              ___   ___   ___

(d)   requires the explicit definition of
target behaviours.

                                              ___   ___   ___

(e)   focuses on the historical determinants
of behaviour.

                                              ___   ___   ___

1.14   Transactional Analysis:

(a)   is associated with Ellis.

                                              ___   ___   ___

(b)   requires the patient to recognise
different Ego-states.

                                              ___   ___   ___

(c)   is also known as assertive training.

                                              ___   ___   ___

(d)   is a brief form of therapy.

                                              ___   ___   ___

(e)   involves "game analysis".

                                              ___   ___   ___

	Ctn	Dbt	Gu

1.15 Cathexis is:

(a) a release of repressed material
accompanied by a release of tension.

(b) a lack of feeling associated with an
emotionally charged subject.

(c) an investment in an object or person
of the psychic energy of a drive.

(d) an element of libido theory.

(e) an uncontrollable urge to perform an
act repeatedly.

**1.16 The following are accurate statements
about defence mechanisims.**

(a) Sigmund Freud produced the first
systematic and comprehensive study of
Ego defences.

(b) Individuals generally have a
characteristic repertoire of defences.

(c) Defences emerge as a result of the Ego's
struggle to mediate between the demands
of the Id and those of reality.

(d) Different defences are associated with
different stages of development.

(e) Reaction formation usually develops in
response to oral impulses.

	Ctn	Dbt	Gu

1.17 The following are contra-indications to E.C.T.

(a) Myocardial infarction twelve months previously.

(b) First trimester of pregnancy.

(c) Raised intracranial pressure.

(d) Old age.

(e) Cardiac pacemaker.

1.18 Features of the "cheese reaction" with monoamine oxidase inhibitors include:

(a) hypotension.

(b) palpitations.

(c) neck stiffness.

(d) acute urinary retention.

(e) sweating.

1.19 Unwanted effects of amitriptyline include:

(a) postural hypotension.

(b) lowering of the epileptic threshold.

(c) withdrawal syndrome after prolonged administration.

(d) diarrhoea.

(e) tremor.

	Ctn	Dbt	Gu

1.20 Lithium carbonate:

(a) is metabolised by the liver.

(b) tends to be retained in patients on diuretics.

(c) has a plasma half-life of less than 8 hours.

(d) is distributed almost solely intracellularly.

(e) reaches peak serum levels 4 to 5 hours after oral administration.

1.21 Benzodiazepines:

(a) facilitate GABA transmission in the CNS.

(b) increase the likelihood of involvement in road traffic accidents.

(c) are more likely to produce side-effects in the elderly.

(d) are commonly fatal in overdose in the elderly.

(e) are contra-indicated in the first trimester of pregnancy.

	Ctn	Dbt	Gu

1.22 In comparison to chlorpromazine, haloperidol:

(a) is less sedative.

(b) is less likely to induce postural hypotension.

(c) is less likely to induce Parkinsonism.

(d) is less likely to induce ECG changes.

(e) is less likely to induce urinary retention.

1.23 Akathisia:

(a) can induce motor overactivity.

(b) is usually experienced as distressing.

(c) occurs in 3 - 5% of patients receiving neuroleptics.

(d) responds temporarily to an increase in the dose of a neuroleptic.

(e) usually responds to amantadine.

	Ctn	Dbt	Gu

1.24 The following statements apply to the epidemiology of senile dementia.

(a) Its incidence rises with increasing age.

(b) Men are more often affected than women.

(c) About 20% of people over 80 are affected.

(d) It is commoner in London than in New York.

(e) Its prevalence is falling in the UK.

1.25 The following are recognised features of Alzheimer's disease.

(a) Increased liability to epilepsy.

(b) Decreased deep tendon reflexes.

(c) Gait disorder.

(d) Aphasia.

(e) Prolixity.

1.26 The following are typical of Korsakov's psychosis.

(a) Impairment of immediate memory.

(b) Fluctuating conscious level.

(c) Retrograde amnesia.

(d) Anterograde amnesia.

(e) Retention of insight.

1.27 Epileptic automatism:

(a) occurs in a state of clear
consciousness.

(b) can occur prior to a seizure.

(c) is always followed by amnesia.

(d) most usually occurs in patients with a
temporal lobe focus.

(e) is a manifestation of hysterical
conversion.

1.28 In neurosyphilis:

(a) urban dwellers are more often affected
than country dwellers.

(b) the lower social classes are more
commonly affected.

(c) the symptoms arise 2 − 5 years after
primary syphilis is contracted.

(d) the sexes are equally affected.

(e) the EEG is usually normal.

	Ctn	Dbt	Gu

1.29   In idiopathic Parkinson's disease:

(a)   euphoria is common.

(b)   lethargy is common.

(c)   depression is usually resistant to
tricyclic antidepressants.

(d)   cognitive impairment occurs in less
than 10% of cases.

(e)   the incidence of dementia is no higher
than in matched controls.

**1.30   Acute intermittent porphyria can be
precipitated by the following drugs.**

(a)   Alcohol.

(b)   Amitriptyline.

(c)   Barbiturates.

(d)   Benzodiazepines.

(e)   Oral contraceptives.

1.31   In Huntington's chorea:

(a)   inheritance is by autosomal recessive
genes.

(b)   suicide rates are increased.

(c)   movement disorders usually precede
psychiatric symptoms.

(d)   the onset may occur in childhood.

(e)   the movement disorders may respond to
haloperidol.

	Ctn	Dbt	Gu

1.32 The lifetime risk of suffering a schizophrenic illness:

(a) is increased in immigrants.

(b) is between 3 and 4% in the UK.

(c) is higher in women than in men.

(d) is highest in the children of social class 5 parents.

(e) is raised in children born in the UK in the first four months of the year.

1.33 The first rank symptoms of schizophrenia:

(a) were first described by Kraepelin.

(b) must be present to make a diagnosis of schizophrenia in accordance with the International Classification of Diseases, Ninth Revision.

(c) do not occur in mania.

(d) indicate a poor prognosis when present in acute schizophrenia.

(e) are all indicative of a breakdown in ego boundaries.

	Ctn	Dbt	Gu

1.34 The following statements apply to catatonic schizophrenia.

(a) Stereotyped movements are common.

(b) ECT is usually of minimal benefit.

(c) Its onset is typically later than in the other sub-types of schizophrenia.

(d) Its incidence has declined in the UK over the last 50 years.

(e) The "psychological pillow" phenomenon may be observed.

1.35 The following behaviours of a family towards their schizophrenic relative have been shown to affect prognosis adversely.

(a) Double-binding.

(b) Projective identification.

(c) Schismatic parenting.

(d) Emotional over-involvement.

(e) High rates of critical comments.

1.36 Cotard's syndrome:

(a)   usually begins in adolescence.   ___   ___   ___

(b)   affects females more often than males. ___   ___   ___

(c)   is frequently associated with depressive
      illness.   ___   ___   ___

(d)   involves nihilistic delusions.   ___   ___   ___

(e)   involves the delusion of doubles.   ___   ___   ___

**1.37 "Secondary mania" occurs as a result
of the following conditions.**

(a)   Viral encephalitis.   ___   ___   ___

(b)   Hypothyroidism.   ___   ___   ___

(c)   Hyperthyroidism.   ___   ___   ___

(d)   Subarachnoid haemorrhage.   ___   ___   ___

(e)   Down's syndrome.   ___   ___   ___

17

	Ctn	Dbt	Gu

1.38 The following statements are true of the epidemiology of depression.

(a) Depression is becoming less common.

(b) The lifetime risk of developing depression is the same for both sexes.

(c) Depression occurring in the menopausal years has a distinct clinical picture.

(d) Depressive symptoms are more common in the divorced than in the married.

(e) Depressive symptoms are most common in social class I.

1.39 The following are typical features of puerperal psychosis.

(a) Dysmorphophobia.

(b) Paranoid delusions.

(c) Perplexity.

(d) Disorientation.

(e) Lability of mood.

	Ctn	Dbt	Gu

1.40 Compared to successful suicide, parasuicide is associated with:

(a) low social class.

(b) depressive illness.

(c) female sex.

(d) seasonal variation.

(e) middle age.

1.41 The following are associated with Seligman's model of depression.

(a) Anaclitic depression.

(b) The apparent independence of reinforcement and behaviour.

(c) Double-binding.

(d) "Vulnerability factors".

(e) Learned helplessness.

1.42 Obsessional neurosis:

(a) is more common among males than females.

(b) is one of the most common neuroses.

(c) usually begins in childhood.

(d) responds well to E.C.T.

(e) represents a regression to a pregenital stage of development, according to Freudian theory.

	Ctn	Dbt	Gu

1.43 Hypochondriacal neurosis:

(a) is a predominantly female disorder.

(b) shows a social class bias.

(c) is most likely to occur in early adulthood.

(d) has a very poor prognosis even with early diagnosis.

(e) is usually secondary to disturbed interpersonal relationships.

1.44 The following are accurate statements about conversion hysteria.

(a) Its presentation varies from culture to culture.

(b) "La belle indifférence" is one of its universal features.

(c) It usually has a gradual onset.

(d) It is synonymous with Briquet's syndrome.

(e) It affects the left of the body more often than the right.

	Ctn	Dbt	Gu

1.45 Features of the hyperventilation syndrome include:

(a) vertigo.

(b) derealization.

(c) chest pain.

(d) tingling in the extremities.

(e) blurred vision.

1.46 Anorexia nervosa:

(a) was first described by Janet.

(b) is 2 - 3 times as common in females as in males.

(c) is probably becoming more common.

(d) has a raised incidence in ballerinas.

(e) occurs most commonly in the lower social classes.

1.47 Good prognostic indicators in anorexia nervosa include:

(a) male sex.

(b) late age at menarche.

(c) short duration of illness prior to treatment.

(d) being married at the time of presentation.

(e) extreme weight loss at the time of presentation.

	Ctn	Dbt	Gu

1.48   The behavioural treatment of obesity:

(a)   emphasises the importance of gratifying repressed oral wishes.

(b)   usually involves aversion therapy.

(c)   usually involves self-monitoring.

(d)   usually involves restriction of exposure to food-related cues.

(e)   has a relapse rate of 5 - 10%.

1.49   The following occur with increased frequency in psychopathic (antisocial) personality disorder.

(a)   Parasuicide.

(b)   Paranoid psychosis.

(c)   Depressive psychosis.

(d)   Drug abuse.

(e)   Alcoholism.

	Ctn	Dbt	Gu

1.50 Delusional mood:

(a) is most usually associated with
schizophrenia.

(b) describes the affect produced by a
specific delusion.

(c) is a derealisation experience.

(d) often precedes the occurrence of
specific delusions.

(e) accounts for the emotional lability
in mania.

1.51 Type A behaviour:

(a) is associated with competitive striving.

(b) can be measured by the Framingham Scale.

(c) cannot be modified by cognitive
behavioural treatment.

(d) is associated with slowly aroused
hostility.

(e) has been shown to be correlated with
neuroticism.

	Ctn	Dbt	Gu

1.52 The Ganser syndrome includes:

(a) hallucinations.

(b) Vorbeireden (approximate answers).

(c) nihilistic delusions.

(d) clouding of consciousness.

(e) glossolalia.

1.53 Masters and Johnson employ the following concepts.

(a) Resolution.

(b) Marital schism.

(c) Plateau.

(d) Orgone.

(e) Sensate focus.

1.54 The symptoms of alcohol withdrawal:

(a) usually start 36 to 48 hours after stopping drinking.

(b) cannot occur while the patient continues to drink.

(c) include auditory hallucinations.

(d) include drowsiness.

(e) usually respond to thiamine.

	Ctn	Dbt	Gu

1.55 In alcoholism, specific benefit has generaly been shown to result from:

(a) psychodynamic psychotherapy. ___ ___ ___

(b) in-patient rather than out-patient treatment. ___ ___ ___

(c) aversion therapy. ___ ___ ___

(d) behaviour therapy. ___ ___ ___

(e) marital stability. ___ ___ ___

1.56 The following drugs are known to give rise to physical dependence.

(a) Barbiturates. ___ ___ ___

(b) Diazepam. ___ ___ ___

(c) Lysergic acid diethylamide (LSD). ___ ___ ___

(d) Cocaine. ___ ___ ___

(e) Morphine. ___ ___ ___

1.57 Solvent abuse:

(a) occurs more frequently in boys than in girls. ___ ___ ___

(b) has a peak incidence in the early teens. ___ ___ ___

(c) is usually a solitary activity. ___ ___ ___

(d) is usually short-lived. ___ ___ ___

(e) frequently leads to physical dependence. ___ ___ ___

	Ctn	Dbt	Gu

1.58 A patient is considered to have "testamentary capacity" (i.e. to be of "sound disposing mind") if he:

(a) knows the nature of his property.

(b) is not deluded.

(c) can assess claims on his property.

(d) understands what a will is.

(e) knows right from wrong.

1.59 The following statements are correct.

(a) The McNaughten Rules were introduced into Scots Law in the mid – 19th Century.

(b) Young delinquents tend to be extraverted ectomorphs.

(c) The incidence of men with an XYY karyotype entering penal institutions confirms there is a significant genetic factor underlying criminal behaviour.

(d) Of those receiving hospital orders in the UK the mentally subnormal are less likely to be reconvicted than the mentally ill.

(e) Epileptics have a higher rate of criminal activity than the general population.

Ctn	Dbt	Gu

1.60 The following are correctly linked with the treatments they introduced.

(a) Delay and Deniker: chlorpromazine.

(b) Cade: electroconvulsive therapy.

(c) Jones: therapeutic community.

(d) Sakel: psychodrama.

(e) Moniz: psychosurgery.

PAPER 2

	Ctn	Dbt	Gu

2.1 Children with specific reading retardation:

(a) are more often girls than boys.

(b) tend to have lower performance than verbal IQs.

(c) are more often left-handed than right-handed.

(d) show increased rates of delinquency.

(e) can usually spell normally.

2.2 Nocturnal enuresis:

(a) is equally common in boys and girls.

(b) in boys is rarely due to urinary tract infection.

(c) shows higher concordance among monozygotic than dizygotic twins.

(d) has a high prevalence among institutionalized children.

(e) is due to excessively rigid toilet training.

		Ctn	Dbt	Gu

2.3 In adolescence:

(a) circumscribed phobic states are more
common than anxiety states.

(b) the prevalence of psychosis is less
than 1 in 1,000.

(c) obsessive – compulsive disorders are
more common than in childhood.

(d) social phobias are more common than in
prepubertal children.

(e) male and female rates for affective
disorders are equal.

2.4 Adjustment reactions in children:

(a) are relatively short-lived.

(b) occur without any apparent pre-existing
mental disorder.

(c) are closely related in time to stress.

(d) are likely to be followed by significant
problems of development.

(e) include specific motor retardation.

	Ctn	Dbt	Gu

2.5 The following statements are correct.

(a) The children of parents with criminal backgrounds have a raised incidence of hyperkinesis.

(b) Schizophrenic parents are likely to have autistic children.

(c) Institutional upbringing from infancy is associated with indiscriminate friendliness.

(d) Emotional disorder is more likely in children from large families.

(e) Marital discord is likely to lead to emotional disturbance in the children.

2.6 Stuttering:

(a) is associated with brain damage.

(b) is more common among those with high generalized anxiety.

(c) is several times more common in left-handed children.

(d) becomes a persistent problem in about 1% of children.

(e) usually begins after 8 years of age.

	Ctn	Dbt	Gu

2.7 The following are common features of early childhood autism.

(a) Increased babbling.

(b) Echolalia.

(c) Impaired language acquisition.

(d) Gaze avoidance.

(e) Ritualistic behaviour.

2.8 The common features of Klinefelter's syndrome include:

(a) abnormalities of the external genitalia.

(b) above average height.

(c) severe subnormality.

(d) increased risk of psychiatric disorder.

(e) aggressiveness.

2.9 Patients with Down's syndrome (trisomy 21):

(a) are more likely to have older mothers than are normal children.

(b) have a single transverse palmar crease.

(c) are likely to be of short stature.

(d) frequently suffer from autism.

(e) suffer from congenital cardiac disorders in about one-third of cases.

	Ctn	Dbt	Gu

2.10 The following conditions result in mental handicap in over 50% of affected children.

(a) Down's syndrome.

(b) Turner's syndrome.

(c) Cri du chat syndrome.

(d) Neurofibromatosis

(e) Hurler's disease.

2.11 Rogerian client-centered therapy emphasizes:

(a) the use of paradoxical intention.

(b) the client's capacity for self-actualization.

(c) the irrational and unsocialized nature of man.

(d) the therapist's empathy and genuineness.

(e) the use of dereflection.

		Ctn	Dbt	Gu

2.12   The main effects of modelling include:

(a)   covert sensitization.   ___ ___ ___

(b)   the acquisition of new response patterns
by the observer.   ___ ___ ___

(c)   the disinhibition of avoided behaviour.   ___ ___ ___

(d)   the facilitation of previously learned
responses.   ___ ___ ___

(e)   the facilitation of insight into the
connection between neutral stimuli and
unconscious wishes.   ___ ___ ___

2.13   The following are associated with Jung.

(a)   The "shadow".   ___ ___ ___

(b)   The "action self".   ___ ___ ___

(c)   A "life style".   ___ ___ ___

(d)   The "orgone".   ___ ___ ___

(e)   The "anima".   ___ ___ ___

	Ctn	Dbt	Gu

2.14 A "corrective emotional experience":

(a) helps undo the damage created by
previous unpleasant experiences.

(b) enables the patient to deal with
unpleasant emotional situations which
previously he would have found
difficult.

(c) is a Jungian concept.

(d) can only take place in the therapeutic
relationship.

(e) helps the patient to become aware of
the irrationality of his emotional
reactions.

2.15 Token economies:

(a) are based on the principles of
classical conditioning.

(b) are means of modifying behaviour in
institutions.

(c) involve strengthening stimulus-response
associations by following the desired
response with a reinforcing stimulus.

(d) are associated with Maxwell Jones.

(e) are associated with Ayllon and Azrin.

	Ctn	Dbt	Gu

2.16 Primal therapy:

(a) was introduced by Perls.

(b) places an emphasis on the recapture of specific childhood memories.

(c) emphasizes the pain of infantile emotional traumas.

(d) focuses on insight as the main aim of therapy.

(e) involves Primary Mental Abilities.

2.17 Memory impairment after E.C.T.:

(a) is often permanent.

(b) can be readily distinguished from memory impairment due to depression.

(c) can include retrograde amnesia for remote events.

(d) often includes impaired learning ability for a few days after treatment.

(e) is probably a product of the anaesthetic agents employed.

2.18 Diazepam:

(a) has an almost immediate effect after
     intramuscular injection.   ___   ___   ___

(b) has, together with its active
     metabolites, a plasma half-life of
     12 – 18 hours.   ___   ___   ___

(c) is metabolised to oxazepam.   ___   ___   ___

(d) induces liver enzyme production.   ___   ___   ___

(e) induces higher plasma levels in the
     elderly after a standard oral dose.   ___   ___   ___

2.19 Mianserin:

(a) is a tricyclic antidepressant.   ___   ___   ___

(b) is a potent histamine antagonist.   ___   ___   ___

(c) has been shown consistently to have a
     weaker antidepressant effect than
     amitriptyline.   ___   ___   ___

(d) causes a widening of the QRS complex.   ___   ___   ___

(e) is safer than amitriptyline in overdose. ___   ___   ___

2.20 Tricyclic antidepressants should not usually be prescribed:

(a) to patients with bundle branch block.   ___   ___   ___

(b) within a month of a myocardial infarction.   ___   ___   ___

(c) in combination with tranylcypromine.   ___   ___   ___

(d) in combination with sulpiride.   ___   ___   ___

(e) to patients with Irritable Bowel syndrome.   ___   ___   ___

2.21 L-tryptophan:

(a) is a precursor of 5-hydroxytryptamine.   ___   ___   ___

(b) is safe in overdose.   ___   ___   ___

(c) can exacerbate the unwanted effects of monoamine oxidase inhibitors.   ___   ___   ___

(d) competes with oestrogen for the same binding sites in plasma.   ___   ___   ___

(e) has no sedative properties.   ___   ___   ___

	Ctn	Dbt	Gu

2.22 Pimozide:

(a) has a plasma half-life of over 36 hours. ___   ___   ___

(b) is a butyrophenone. ___   ___   ___

(c) produces less sedation than chlorpromazine. ___   ___   ___

(d) produces fewer anticholinergic side-effects than chlorpromazine. ___   ___   ___

(e) produces minimal Parkinsonian side-effects. ___   ___   ___

2.23 In patients treated with neuroleptic drugs, akathisia:

(a) occurs later in treatment than Parkinsonian side-effects. ___   ___   ___

(b) occurs more often in men than in women. ___   ___   ___

(c) probably results from an underlying psychosis. ___   ___   ___

(d) is usually alleviated by anti-cholinergic drugs. ___   ___   ___

(e) is more common in the elderly. ___   ___   ___

	Ctn	Dbt	Gu

2.24 In late paraphrenia:

(a) paranoid symptoms are common.

(b) auditory hallucinations are common.

(c) the premorbid personality is usually normal.

(d) depressive symptoms rarely occur.

(e) ECT is usually the treatment of choice.

2.25 Multi-infarct dementia:

(a) is commonly associated with hypertension.

(b) accounts for less than 30% of senile dementias.

(c) tends to develop at a later age than senile dementia of the Alzheimer type (SDAT).

(d) is more commonly associated with emotional lability than is SDAT.

(e) is more common than SDAT in men under 75 years.

	Ctn	Dbt	Gu

2.26 The degree of intellectual impairment after penetrating head injuries:

(a) is closely related to the length of post-traumatic amnesia.

(b) is usually greater than after non-penetrating head injuries.

(c) is usually greater with left rather than right hemispheric lesions.

(d) is greatest when the temporal lobe is affected.

(e) is unrelated to the amount of brain damage.

2.27 Creutzfeld – Jakob disease:

(a) is inherited by an X-linked recessive gene.

(b) is characterised by nihilistic delusions.

(c) usually has an insidious onset.

(d) usually worsens rapidly.

(e) probably results from aluminium toxicity.

	Ctn	Dbt	Gu

2.28 Auras associated with temporal lobe epilepsy include:

(a) jamais vu.

(b) olfactory hallucinations.

(c) epigastric sensations.

(d) anxiety.

(e) visual hallucinations.

2.29 In "myxoedematous madness":

(a) the EEG is usually slowed.

(b) cerebral blood flow is decreased.

(c) symptoms always develop insidiously.

(d) cognitive impairment is unusual.

(e) paranoid symptoms are characteristic.

2.30 In Wernicke's encephalopathy:

(a) the majority, if untreated, develop a Korsakov's syndrome.

(b) the white matter of the brain is principally affected.

(c) the mamillary bodies are damaged.

(d) intravenous thiamine should be delayed until electrolyte balance has been achieved.

(e) nystagmus usually recovers before ophthalmoplegias.

	Ctn	Dbt	Gu

2.31 Tardive dyskinesia:

(a) usually arises within the first six
     months of treatment with neuroleptics.

(b) is intensified during sleep.

(c) is intensified by anxiety.

(d) most commonly affects the face and
     tongue.

(e) does not occur before puberty.

**2.32 In a young man suffering his first
       schizophrenic illness, the following
       indicate a better than average prognosis.**

(a) High IQ.

(b) Acute onset.

(c) The presence of guilt feelings.

(d) Single status.

(e) Family history of depressive illness.

	Ctn	Dbt	Gu

2.33   In schizophrenia, the 'drift hypothesis':

(a)   helps to explain schizophrenic thought disorder.

(b)   can be supported by testing with the Repertory Grid.

(c)   helps to explain the disparity in social class between schizophrenics and their fathers.

(d)   helps to explain the high concentration of schizophrenics in inner city areas.

(e)   helps to explain the genetic transmission of the disorder.

2.34   The following are considered characteristic of schizophrenic thought disorder.

(a)   Circumstantiality.

(b)   Thought alienation.

(c)   Primary process thinking.

(d)   Perseveration.

(e)   Asyndesis.

	Ctn	Dbt	Gu

2.35 In schizophrenia, life events:

(a) precipitate relapse but have no effect in precipitating first illnesses.   ___ ___ ___

(b) have minimal effect on the course of the illness.   ___ ___ ___

(c) have no effect on the course of the illness when the event is favourable.   ___ ___ ___

(d) have been shown to be of importance only in males.   ___ ___ ___

(e) have no effect on the course of the illness when patients live in low expressed emotion families.   ___ ___ ___

2.36 The following features in a psychotic parent increase the likelihood of his fathering a psychotic child.

(a) Psychotic illness in his wife's family.   ___ ___ ___

(b) Psychotic illness in other first-degree relatives.   ___ ___ ___

(c) Mixed hemisphere dominance.   ___ ___ ___

(d) Onset of illness late in life.   ___ ___ ___

(e) Evidence of organic aetiology.   ___ ___ ___

	Ctn	Dbt	Gu

2.37 The following are features of delusional depression.

(a) Nihilistic delusions.

(b) Hypochondriacal delusions.

(c) Grandiose delusions.

(d) Delusions of persecution.

(e) Delusions of passivity.

2.38 Depressed patients:

(a) have increased E scores on the Eysenck Personality Inventory (EPI).

(b) have increased N scores on the EPI.

(c) have very similar scores on the EPI when ill and when recovered.

(d) tend to be extrapunitive.

(e) tend to direct aggression progressively outward as they recover.

	Ctn	Dbt	Gu

2.39 Following a stillbirth:

(a) the mother should be sedated with
neuroleptics.   ___ ___ ___

(b) it is usually helpful to encourage the
mother to hold the dead baby.   ___ ___ ___

(c) the mother should be encouraged to
become pregnant again as quickly as
possible.   ___ ___ ___

(d) the mother usually experiences a grief
reaction.   ___ ___ ___

(e) a future child may be a victim of the
"replacement child syndrome".   ___ ___ ___

2.40 Suicide rates in the UK:

(a) have increased in the period
1975 to 1980.   ___ ___ ___

(b) are higher in winter than in spring.   ___ ___ ___

(c) are higher in rural than in urban areas. ___ ___ ___

(d) are inversely related to homicide rates. ___ ___ ___

(e) are similar for male and female
depressives.   ___ ___ ___

	Ctn	Dbt	Gu

2.41 **In the bereaved, the following features increase the likelihood of a poor outcome.**

(a) Excessive self-reproach.

(b) Previous mental illness.

(c) Physical illness.

(d) Previous unresolved losses.

(e) Unemployment.

2.42 **Agoraphobia:**

(a) occurs with equal frequency in both sexes.

(b) is usually associated with marital disharmony.

(c) generally remits spontaneously more quickly than anxiety states.

(d) usually develops between 35 and 50 years of age.

(e) has as its most prominent feature a fear of open spaces.

	Ctn	Dbt	Gu

2.43 Obsessions:

(a) are usually unacceptable to the patient.

(b) are stereotyped acts.

(c) generally produce distress for the patient.

(d) respond well to interpretive psychotherapy.

(e) rarely involve aggressive material.

2.44 The psychoanalytic theory of hysteria states that:

(a) the symptom represents omnipotence of thought.

(b) regression is the principal underlying defence.

(c) there are sexual conflicts originating in the Oedipal stage of development.

(d) the energy from the sexual drive is translated into a physical symptom.

(e) secondary gain arises from the resolution of the unconscious conflict underlying symptom formation.

	Ctn	Dbt	Gu

2.45 "Compensation neuroses" are:

(a) unrelated to the degree of injury.

(b) resolved once compensation has been obtained.

(c) ten times more likely in men than in women.

(d) more common in younger individuals.

(e) more common among the poorly educated.

2.46 In anorexia nervosa:

(a) menstrual dysfunction occurs only after significant weight loss.

(b) menorrhagia is relatively common.

(c) increased libido is relatively common.

(d) gonadotrophin levels are usually reduced.

(e) testosterone levels are usually reduced in males.

49

	Ctn	Dbt	Gu

2.47 Studies of the families of patients with anorexia nervosa have shown that:

(a) concordance is higher for monozygotic than for dizygotic twins. ___ ___ ___

(b) siblings have an increased risk of the disorder. ___ ___ ___

(c) relatives have increased rates of alcoholism. ___ ___ ___

(d) relatives have increased rates of affective disorder. ___ ___ ___

(e) relatives have increased rates of presenile dementia. ___ ___ ___

2.48 Adequately controlled trials have shown bulimia nervosa to respond to:

(a) sulpiride. ___ ___ ___

(b) chlorpromazine. ___ ___ ___

(c) phenelzine. ___ ___ ___

(d) ECT. ___ ___ ___

(e) imipramine. ___ ___ ___

	Ctn	Dbt	Gu

2.49 Munchausen syndrome:

(a) was first described by Asher.

(b) is essentially a depressive illness.

(c) has also been called the "Hospital
      Addiction Syndrome".

(d) is the same as dysmorphophobia.

(e) is resistant to treatment.

**2.50 Idiopathic narcolepsy is associated
        with:**

(a) cataplexy.

(b) sleep paralysis.

(c) increased likelihood of road
      traffic accidents.

(d) absence of paradoxical sleep.

(e) onset in middle age.

2.51 Autoscopy:

(a) is the same as "phantom mirror-image".

(b) occurs in normal people.

(c) is almost always a hysterical symptom.

(d) occurs in epilepsy.

(e) occurs in toxic confusional states.

	Ctn	Dbt	Gu

2.52 Hospital admission rates are increasing for women in the UK in the following diagnostic categories.

(a) Schizophrenia.

(b) Depressive neurosis.

(c) Depressive psychosis.

(d) Alcoholism.

(e) Senile dementia.

2.53 Homosexuality:

(a) is probably not as widespread in the UK as was implied by the work of Kinsey.

(b) in our culture is no more likely than heterosexuality to be associated with psychological problems.

(c) is commonly associated with sexual violence.

(d) is best dealt with by aversion therapy.

(e) may be potentiated by foetal hormonal abnormalities.

| | Ctn | Dbt | Gu |

2.54 Alcohol related problems occur:

(a) in 2 - 5% of medical in-patients.

(b) in men more often than in women.

(c) most commonly in the middle
socio-economic groups.

(d) more commonly in Protestants than
in Roman Catholics.

(e) more commonly in urban than in rural
dwellers.

2.55 Delirium tremens:

(a) has a mortality rate of over 5%.

(b) occurs in about 30% of alcoholic
in-patients.

(c) usually continues for 5 to 7 days.

(d) should be treated in a darkened room.

(e) is associated with respiratory
alkalosis.

**2.56 Cannabis abuse is known to be
associated with:**

(a) auditory hallucinations.

(b) visual hallucinations.

(c) paranoid delusions.

(d) brain damage.

(e) hepatic necrosis.

	Ctn	Dbt	Gu

2.57 Symptoms of opiate withdrawal include:

(a) diarrhoea. — — —

(b) piloerection. — — —

(c) perspiration. — — —

(d) lacrimation. — — —

(e) rhinorrhoea. — — —

2.58 Incest:

(a) can occur without sexual intercourse. — — —

(b) was rarely reported by males in
Kinsey's studies. — — —

(c) is more likly between siblings than
between parents and offspring. — — —

(d) occurs mainly in the lower socio-
economic groups. — — —

(e) is more likely to be committed by those
of higher intelligence compared to other
sexual offenders. — — —

	Ctn	Dbt	Gu

2.59 Exhibitionism:

(a) in older age groups suggests a major psychiatric disorder.

(b) is generally a recurring offence.

(c) is commonly associated with violent sexual acts against children.

(d) may also be called "scopophilia".

(e) is associated with low IQ.

2.60 The following individuals advocated a humane approach to the mentally disturbed.

(a) Sprenger.

(b) Esquirol.

(c) Dix.

(d) Pinel.

(e) Willis.

PAPER 3

	Ctn	Dbt	Gu

3.1 Faecal soiling:

(a) occurs in 1-2% of 7 year olds.

(b) is more common in boys than in girls.

(c) has a positive association with enuresis.

(d) has a positive association with large family size.

(e) is considered abnormal if it occurs after 2 years of age.

3.2 In "non-organic failure to thrive":

(a) head circumference is characteristically reduced.

(b) weight is below the 3rd percentile.

(c) there has frequently been an initial maladaptive parent-child relationship.

(d) the child typically prefers to play with inanimate toys.

(e) the child is at increased risk of parental abuse.

	Ctn	Dbt	Gu

3.3 In Gilles de la Tourette's syndrome:

(a) there is usually an emotional
precipitant.

(b) nearly half of those affected have
schizoid personalities.

(c) inheritance is by X-linked recessive
genes.

(d) the EEG is diagnostic.

(e) abnormal movements decrease during
sleep.

3.4 In children, conversion hysteria:

(a) is equally common in boys and girls.

(b) is becoming less common.

(c) may develop through identification.

(d) is usually accompanied by conduct
disorder.

(e) is usually accompanied by anxiety.

**3.5 A poor prognosis for behavioural
difficulties in pre-school children is
made more likely by:**

(a) early language delay.

(b) marital disharmony between the parents.

(c) maternal depression.

(d) female sex of the child.

(e) developmental delay.

	Ctn	Dbt	Gu

3.6 School refusal:

(a) shows a male: female preponderance of 2:1.

(b) is more common among the lower social classes.

(c) is more likely in children from broken homes.

(d) is more common among only children.

(e) occurs in about 25% of psychiatrically disturbed children.

3.7 The "Fragile X" syndrome:

(a) can be diagnosed in utero.

(b) does not occur in normal males.

(c) is also known as the Martin-Bell-Renpenning syndrome.

(d) occurs in about 1 per 100,000 of the general population.

(e) is rarely associated with a speech impediment.

	Ctn	Dbt	Gu

3.8 The following causes of mental handicap are inherited as X-linked recessive genes.

(a) Tay-Sachs' disease.

(b) Phenylketonuria.

(c) Lesch-Nyhan syndrome.

(d) Tuberous sclerosis.

(e) Neurofibromatosis.

3.9 Hyperkinesis in mentally handicapped patients:

(a) should always be treated with methylphenidate or dexamphetamine.

(b) is more likely if they are also epileptic.

(c) is particularly common in those with only mild degrees of handicap.

(d) is associated with characteristic EEG abnormalities.

(e) is commonly due to an underlying manic-depressive psychosis.

	Ctn	Dbt	Gu

3.10 Principal features of the Lesch-Nyhan syndrome include:

(a) self-mutilatory behaviour.

(b) choreoathetosis.

(c) headbanging.

(d) hyperuricaemia.

(e) severe intellectual impairment.

3.11 Aversion therapy:

(a) includes response prevention.

(b) should not be used with children.

(c) involves linking unwanted behaviour with responses usually associated with aversive stimuli.

(d) includes response cost.

(e) includes flooding.

	Ctn	Dbt	Gu

3.12 The claims of traditional Freudian theory include the following.

(a) The manifest content of dreams refers to the material which the therapist seeks to reveal by means of interpretation.

(b) The features of secondary process thinking are characteristic of the latent content of dreams.

(c) The Super-ego prevents the fulfilment of the Ego-ideal.

(d) "Dream work" is the patient's effort to reveal the latent content of dreams.

(e) The "latency period" marks a resurgence of the sexual drive.

3.13 Gestalt therapy:

(a) was devised by Perls.

(b) emphasizes the responsibility of the individual for his own situation.

(c) emphasizes the value of interpretation even more than does psychodynamic therapy.

(d) has as its hallmark prescriptive techniques.

(e) views the therapeutic encounter as a recreation of past significant relationships.

	Ctn	Dbt	Gu

3.14 Reality testing:

(a) refers to the Ego's capacity for
objective evaluation of the world.

(b) begins to develop in childhood.

(c) conforms to the Pleasure Principle.

(d) leads to the development of
transference.

(e) becomes impaired when regression occurs.

**3.15 The following have contributed
specifically to developments in Crisis
Theory.**

(a) Kübler-Ross.

(b) Thomas.

(c) Caplan.

(d) Brandon.

(e) Bannister.

	Ctn	Dbt	Gu

3.16 Implosive therapy:

(a) was devised by Wolpe.

(b) involves the patient imagining anxiety-
provoking stimuli.

(c) is designed to eliminate avoidance
behaviour.

(d) requires anxiety to be experienced
without any actual adverse consequences.

(e) requires the patient to interupt a train
of thought by a sudden distracting
stimulus.

3.17 Electroconvulsive therapy:

(a) has been in use in the UK for over 40
years.

(b) is of proven effectiveness in psychotic
depression.

(c) is of proven effectiveness in severe
hypochondriacal neurosis.

(d) is of proven effectiveness in chronic
schizophrenia.

(e) exerts a synergistic effect with
antidepressants in the treatment of
severe depression.

	Ctn	Dbt	Gu

3.18 Physiological changes which occur after ECT include:

(a) EEG changes which usually persist for over a week.

(b) a rise in serum prolactin shortly after the treatment.

(c) a fall in plasma cortisol within an hour of the treatment.

(d) an initial bradycardia and subsequent tachycardia.

(e) a decrease in cerebral circulation.

3.19 On account of their high tyramine content, the following foodstuffs should not be taken in combination with monoamine oxidase inhibitors.

(a) Salmon.

(b) Stilton cheese.

(c) Bovril.

(d) Broad bean pods.

(e) Cottage cheese.

| | Ctn | Dbt | Gu |

3.20 Cardiovascular effects of amitriptyline include:

(a) tachycardia.

(b) sudden cardiac death.

(c) antagonism of the anti-hypertensive effect of methyldopa.

(d) postural hypotension.

(e) cardiac arrhythmias.

3.21 The symptoms of lithium toxicity:

(a) do not occur until blood levels exceed 1.3 m.mol/l.

(b) tend to occur at lower blood levels in the elderly.

(c) include constipation.

(d) include nystagmus.

(e) include oliguria.

3.22 Nitrazepam:

(a) has muscle relaxant properties.

(b) has a plasma half-life of less than 12 hours.

(c) induces few "hang-over" effects when used as a hypnotic.

(d) has greater effects on psychomotor performance than clobazam.

(e) has anti-epileptic properties.

	Ctn	Dbt	Gu

3.23 The symptoms/signs of neuroleptic-induced Parkinsonism include:

(a) bradykinesia.

(b) hypersalivation.

(c) choreiform movements.

(d) tremor.

(e) micrographia.

3.24 In depressive pseudodementia:

(a) senile dementia usually develops.

(b) about 0.5% of elderly depressives are affected.

(c) the patient seldom complains of memory impairment.

(d) "don't know" answers are characteristic.

(e) there is often a previous history of depression.

3.25 The following are more likely to occur in multi-infarct dementia than in senile dementia of the Alzheimer type.

(a) Acute onset.

(b) Nocturnal confusion.

(c) Urinary incontinence.

(d) Personality deterioration.

(e) Depression.

	Ctn	Dbt	Gu

3.26 Typical features of subdural haematoma include:

(a) headache.

(b) fluctuating conscious level.

(c) normal EEG.

(d) lateral rectus paralysis.

(e) Parkinsonism.

3.27 Epileptic automatism:

(a) is rarely preceded by an aura.

(b) may take the form of stereotyped utterances.

(c) rarely involves an aggressive act.

(d) can occur with frontal lobe foci.

(e) can occur in petit mal epilepsy.

3.28 The following are commonly found in patients with hepatic encephalopathy.

(a) Drowsiness.

(b) Tremor.

(c) Aggression.

(d) Aggravation of symptoms by low protein diet.

(e) EEG abnormalities.

	Ctn	Dbt	Gu

3.29 In neurosyphilis:

(a) serological tests for syphilis may be negative.

(b) depression is common.

(c) affective symptoms are optimally treated with ECT.

(d) dementia is common.

(e) dysarthria is common.

3.30 The following are features of acute intermittent porphyria.

(a) Abdominal pain.

(b) Constipation.

(c) Neuropathies.

(d) Convulsions.

(e) Delirium.

3.31 The following are recognised psychiatric presentations of Huntington's chorea.

(a) Obsessional neurosis.

(b) Hypochondriasis.

(c) Schizophreniform psychosis.

(d) Dementia.

(e) Paranoid psychosis.

	Ctn	Dbt	Gu

**3.32 The following authors have advanced
hypotheses regarding the importance of
patients' family dynamics in
precipitating schizophrenia.**

(a) Kringlen. ___ ___ ___

(b) Lidz. ___ ___ ___

(c) Heston. ___ ___ ___

(d) Fromm-Reichman. ___ ___ ___

(e) Bateson. ___ ___ ___

**3.33 Patients making the following
statements have a first rank symptom
of schizophrenia.**

(a) "I knew the man next to me could hear
what I was thinking." ___ ___ ___

(b) "I heard a voice telling me I was going
to be killed." ___ ___ ___

(c) "I saw the milkman putting down a bottle
and I knew there was going to be a
nuclear war." ___ ___ ___

(d) "It was a strange force inside me that
made me break the window." ___ ___ ___

(e) "I don't seem able to think for myself.
All my thoughts seem to be my mother's." ___ ___ ___

	Ctn	Dbt	Gu

3.34 A viral aetiology of schizophrenia is supported by:

(a) the reported epidemiology of schizophrenia in Papua New Guinea.

(b) the incidence of schizophrenia in psychiatric nurses.

(c) the fertility of schizophrenics.

(d) the seasonal pattern of birthdates in schizophrenics.

(e) adenovirus antibody titres in chronic schizophrenics.

3.35 In chronic schizophrenia, depression:

(a) occurs in 2 - 5% of cases.

(b) is nearly always the result of treatment with depot neuroleptics.

(c) responds readily to tricyclic antidepressants.

(d) varies inversely in severity with extrapyramidal side-effects of neuroleptics.

(e) is precipitated by a life event in over 80% of cases.

70

	Ctn	Dbt	Gu

3.36 The following drugs are known to induce depressive illness.

(a) Clonidine.

(b) Oral contraceptives.

(c) Corticosteroids.

(d) Methyldopa.

(e) Propranolol.

3.37 In hypomania, the following are relatively common.

(a) Transient depressive episodes.

(b) Excessive alcohol consumption.

(c) Euphoria.

(d) Suicide.

(e) Threatening auditory hallucinations.

3.38 Folie à deux:

(a) was first described by Janet.

(b) is a type of schizophrenic thought disorder.

(c) usually starts with an illness in the submissive partner.

(d) most usually occurs in married couples.

(e) usually involves schizophrenia in the dominant partner.

	Ctn	Dbt	Gu

3.39 In the puerperium:

(a) the onset of schizophrenia carries a
good prognosis.

(b) there is no real increase in the
incidence of psychotic illness.

(c) affective symptoms peak in severity on
day 2 post partum.

(d) neurotic depression is the most common
psychiatric illness.

(e) "maternity blues" occur in less than
20% of mothers.

3.40 Research into suicide suggests that:

(a) in the spring there is a more marked
rise in suicides in rural areas than in
urban communities.

(b) at least three quarters of suicides
have at some time suffered from a
mental illness.

(c) at least 50% of suicides have no
previous history of suicidal attempts.

(d) schizophrenia is the second most common
disorder associated with suicide.

(e) an estimated 1 to 2% of parasuicides
kill themselves within a 1 to 2 year
period.

	Ctn	Dbt	Gu

3.41 The differential diagnosis of depressive illness may include the following.

(a) Chronic brucellosis.

(b) Addison's disease.

(c) Phaeochromocytoma.

(d) Hypothyroidism.

(e) Cushing's disease.

3.42 The following are manifestations of hysterical dissociation.

(a) 'Latah'.

(b) Gelineau's syndrome.

(c) Amok.

(d) Capgras' syndrome.

(e) Klüver-Bucy syndrome.

3.43 A phobia:

(a) is out of proportion to the demands of the situation.

(b) can occur in otherwise healthy individuals.

(c) cannot be reasoned away.

(d) is beyond voluntary control.

(e) leads to avoidance of the feared situation.

	Ctn	Dbt	Gu

3.44 Depersonalization:

(a) can occur in multiple sclerosis.

(b) may be induced by sensory deprivation.

(c) may be a form of psychic defence.

(d) commonly occurs in association with agoraphobia.

(e) does not occur in schizophrenia.

3.45 A fugue:

(a) usually has a clearly defined precipitant.

(b) usually lasts for over a week.

(c) occasionally involves behaviour uncharacteristic of the sufferer.

(d) often involves amnesia for the events that occurred during it.

(e) is a dissociated state.

3.46 The following are features of anorexia nervosa.

(a) Hypothermia.

(b) Hypotension.

(c) Hypocholesterolaemia

(d) Hypocarotenaemia.

(e) Hypoglycaemia.

| | Ctn | Dbt | Gu |

3.47 **The following statements apply to the outcome of anorexia nervosa.**

(a) Menstrual function normalises in the majority of cases.

(b) The rate of initial weight gain is the best prognostic indicator.

(c) Mortality rates from the illness are 20 - 30%.

(d) Over 90% of patients maintain normal eating patterns.

(e) Over 90% of patients maintain normal weight.

3.48 **Bulimia nervosa:**

(a) has a prevalence of 1 - 2/1000 women.

(b) does not occur in men.

(c) is usually distressing to the patient.

(d) tends to affect older women than does anorexia nervosa.

(e) is a term introduced by Russell.

	Ctn	Dbt	Gu

3.49 Obsessional personality disorder is characterised by:

(a) violent outbursts.

(b) rigidity.

(c) tidiness.

(d) propensity to develop depressive illness.

(e) propensity to develop paranoid psychosis.

3.50 An excess of "life events" has been demonstrated prior to:

(a) the onset of depressive illness.

(b) the onset of manic illness.

(c) the onset of senile dementia.

(d) appendicectomies.

(e) relapses in schizophrenia.

Ctn   Dbt   Gu

3.51 The "Irritable Bowel" syndrome:

(a) is associated with abdominal pain in
less than 50% of cases.   ___   ___   ___

(b) may be exacerbated by threatening life
events.   ___   ___   ___

(c) is more commonly associated with
neurotic personality features than is
ulcerative colitis.   ___   ___   ___

(d) is equally common among males and
females.   ___   ___   ___

(e) is an inflammatory disorder.   ___   ___   ___

3.52 The following observations are correct.

(a) The victims of indecent exposure are
likely to be at or around the age of
puberty.   ___   ___   ___

(b) Convicted paedophiles rarely have a
preference for children of one sex.   ___   ___   ___

(c) Childhood transsexualism in boys is
more likely to lead to homosexuality
than to transsexualism in adulthood.   ___   ___   ___

(d) Fetishism is equally common in
males and females.   ___   ___   ___

(e) There is a significantly higher
concordance for homosexuality among
monozygotic than dizygotic twins.   ___   ___   ___

| | Ctn | Dbt | Gu |

3.53 In alcoholic hallucinosis:

(a) Schneiderian first rank symptoms are
rare.

(b) visual hallucinations are more common
than auditory hallucinations.

(c) hallucinations may occur while the
patient continues to drink.

(d) hallucinations usually follow an
epileptic fit.

(e) there is usually a strong family
history of schizophrenia.

3.54 Features of alcohol dependence include:

(a) amnesic episodes.

(b) morning nausea.

(c) increased alcohol tolerance.

(d) ataxia.

(e) drinking to avoid withdrawal symptoms.

**3.55 The features of foetal alcohol
syndrome include:**

(a) decreased head circumference.

(b) hypersomnia.

(c) cardiac abnormalities.

(d) maxillary hypoplasia.

(e) blindness.

	Ctn	Dbt	Gu

3.56 The effects of amphetamines include:

(a) increased hunger.

(b) euphoria.

(c) bradycardia.

(d) hypotension.

(e) sweating.

3.57 Solvent abuse is associated with:

(a) impaired scholastic performance.

(b) high rates of neurotic disorder.

(c) cerebellar degeneration.

(d) focal slow wave complexes on EEG.

(e) progression to heroin abuse in
      15-20% of cases.

**3.58 The following statements about
        rape are correct.**

(a) Compared to victims of homicide, rape
      victims are rarely attacked by
      strangers.

(b) The offender and victim usually live
      in the same neighbourhood.

(c) Most rapes are unplanned.

(d) Most rapes occur indoors.

(e) For most victims, depressive symptoms
      resolve within four months.

	Ctn	Dbt	Gu

3.59 The following statements are correct under English Law.

(a) "Diminished responsibility" can be raised only if the charge is murder.

(b) A child of 12 years and over is presumed to be fully responsible.

(c) A child of 9 years is held to be capable of forming a guilty intent if he is able to discern good from evil.

(d) The offence of indecent assault does not require proof of guilty intent.

(e) The offence of murder does not require proof of guilty intent.

3.60 The following individuals and disorders are correctly linked.

(a) Wernicke: neuraesthenia.

(b) Cullen: neurosis.

(c) Morel: démence précoce.

(d) Sydenham: hysteria.

(e) Beard: aphasia.

PAPER 4

	Ctn	Dbt	Gu

4.1 Elective mutism in children:

(a) usually follows a major trauma.

(b) is more common among girls than boys.

(c) is associated with speech delay.

(d) has a good response to treatment.

(e) is often accompanied by behaviour
problems.

4.2 Tics:

(a) are more frequent among girls than
among boys.

(b) cease during sleep.

(c) typically begin between 5 - 10 years.

(d) are associated with low IQ.

(e) usually persist for several years.

	Ctn	Dbt	Gu

4.3 The prevalence of conduct disorder is higher in children:

(a) from white English families than from immigrant West Indian families. ___ ___ ___

(b) with recurrent physical illness. ___ ___ ___

(c) with intellectual retardation. ___ ___ ___

(d) following bereavement. ___ ___ ___

(e) from families with marital discord. ___ ___ ___

4.4 In children, genetic factors have been shown to contribute to the aetiology of:

(a) specific reading retardation. ___ ___ ___

(b) stealing from home. ___ ___ ___

(c) fire-setting. ___ ___ ___

(d) faecal soiling. ___ ___ ___

(e) school refusal. ___ ___ ___

	Ctn	Dbt	Gu

4.5 The following statements apply to childhood enuresis.

(a) It is significantly associated with adverse social factors.

(b) It is significantly associated with conduct disorders.

(c) It is significantly associated with neurotic disorders.

(d) A short course of tricyclic antidepressants is curative in the majority of cases.

(e) Drinking before bedtime can improve outcome with the "buzzer alarm".

4.6 The following statements about adolescence are correct.

(a) Prepubertal adolescents have few heterosexual interests.

(b) Adolescents from single-parent families are likely to have poor self-esteem.

(c) Adolescence is the most common age of onset for anorexia nervosa.

(d) Animal phobias are as likely as social phobias to arise for the first time in adolescence.

(e) Delinquency rises to a peak in the late teens.

| | Ctn | Dbt | Gu |

4.7 Early childhood autism:

(a) is not associated with epilepsy.

(b) was first systematically described by Kanner.

(c) is associated with severe intellectual impairment in over 50% of cases.

(d) can be caused by abnormal parenting.

(e) is more common in boys than in girls.

4.8 The following statements are true of chromosomal abnormalities.

(a) 1 - 1.5/1000 live-born babies show a detectable chromosomal abnormality.

(b) They constitute the commonest genetic cause of mental handicap.

(c) Children with Trisomy 13 tend to be less severely handicapped than those with Down's syndrome.

(d) About a half of foetuses aborting spontaneously before 12 weeks gestation show major chromosomal abnormalities.

(e) Trisomy 18 (Edward's syndrome) is compatible with normal intelligence.

	Ctn	Dbt	Gu

4.9 The following statements are true of Tay-Sach's disease.

(a) It is an infantile form of cerebromacular degeneration.

(b) It is particularly common in North American Indians.

(c) Spasticity is a common feature.

(d) A "cherry red spot" is evident on the macula of the retina.

(e) A "butterfly rash" appears on the face.

4.10 Patients suffering from Down's syndrome:

(a) are particularly prone to Alzheimer's disease in adult life.

(b) are vulnerable to affective disorders in adult life.

(c) are less susceptible to epilepsy in childhood than are autistic children.

(d) usually become more easily managed at home once they reach adolescence.

(e) who display echolalia are suffering from a co-existent psychosis.

	Ctn	Dbt	Gu

4.11 Therapeutic Communities are associated with:

(a) Szasz.

(b) democratic ideals.

(c) reality confrontation.

(d) liberal, humanitarian ideals.

(e) the avoidance of the antitherapeutic effects of institutions.

4.12 Operant conditioning is associated with:

(a) schedules of reinforcement.

(b) behavioural change as a function of change in consequences.

(c) shaping.

(d) Pavlov.

(e) the presentation of reinforcement by the experimenter irrespective of the subject's behaviour.

4.13 The following are attributable to Bion.

(a) The "pairing group".

(b) The "fight/flight group".

(c) The "encounter group".

(d) The "dependency group".

(e) The "T-group".

	Ctn	Dbt	Gu

4.14   Biofeedback:

(a)   is based on the Premack Principle.

(b)   facilitates the voluntary regulation of physiological functions.

(c)   can only be used with physiological processes governed by the autonomic nervous system.

(d)   was devised by Eysenck.

(e)   may involve analogue and binary feedback.

4.15   Abreaction can be triggered by:

(a)   psychodrama.

(b)   hexobarbitone.

(c)   methamphetamine.

(d)   alcohol.

(e)   sudden noises.

4.16   The following are correctly linked.

(a)   Beck: Rational - Emotive therapy.

(b)   Ellis: modelling.

(c)   Skinner: operant conditioning.

(d)   Watson: classical conditioning.

(e)   Wolpe: behavioural therapy by reciprocal inhibition.

	Ctn	Dbt	Gu

4.17 Compared with bilateral treatment, unilateral ECT to the non-dominant hemisphere:

(a) causes less memory impairment.

(b) is less likely to cause post-ECT confusion.

(c) delivers less electrical energy to the brain.

(d) usually requires fewer treatments to achieve the same response.

(e) is less likely to cause headaches.

4.18 The symptoms of benzodiazepine withdrawal syndrome include:

(a) insomnia.

(b) tremor.

(c) drowsiness.

(d) epileptic fits.

(e) headache.

	Ctn	Dbt	Gu

4.19 Imipramine:

(a) is a potent inhibitor of 5-HT re-uptake.

(b) is a potent inhibitor of noradrenaline re-uptake.

(c) is less sedative than amitriptyline.

(d) is less sedative than doxepin.

(e) causes more anticholinergic side-effects than doxepin.

4.20 L-tryptophan:

(a) has a plasma half-life of 18 - 24 hours.

(b) is a naturally occurring amino-acid.

(c) should not be given in combination with tricyclic antidepressants.

(d) causes a rise in CSF 5-hydroxy-indole-acetic acid when taken orally.

(e) decreases re-uptake of noradrenaline.

4.21 Lithium carbonate:

(a) was first used on psychiatric patients by Schou.

(b) inhibits the formation of cyclic AMP.

(c) is of proven efficacy in the prophylaxis of bipolar affective disorder.

(d) is safe during pregnancy.

(e) is secreted in breast milk.

	Ctn	Dbt	Gu

4.22 Unwanted effects of chlorpromazine include:

(a) photosensitivity.

(b) retinitis pigmentosa.

(c) leucopenia.

(d) urticaria.

(e) polycythemia.

4.23 Thioridazine:

(a) is a thioxanthene.

(b) is minimally sedative.

(c) causes fewer Parkinsonian side-effects than chlorpromazine.

(d) has minimal anti-cholinergic properties.

(e) lowers serum prolactin levels.

4.24 In the elderly, neurotic illnesses:

(a) increase in prevalence with increasing age.

(b) are more common than at any other time of adult life.

(c) affect the sexes equally.

(d) are most commonly depressive neuroses.

(e) have arisen before the age of 50 in over 80% of cases.

90

| | Ctn | Dbt | Gu |

4.25 The demented elderly:

(a) show an increased likelihood of having a demented sibling.

(b) have a similar life expectancy to the non-demented elderly.

(c) are now surviving for a shorter time after entering longterm hospital care.

(d) are usually in institutional care.

(e) are most likely to require institutional care if they live with a married daughter.

4.26 In presenile dementia, the following early features are suggestive of Pick's disease.

(a) Dysphasia.

(b) Dyspraxia.

(c) Personality changes.

(d) Agnosia.

(e) Incontinence.

	Ctn	Dbt	Gu

4.27   In grand mal epilepsy:

(a)   women are more often affected than men.

(b)   monozygotic twins are more often both affected than are dizygotic twins.

(c)   suicide rates are increased.

(d)   cerebral tumours are the cause in over 50% of cases when the onset is after age 25 years.

(e)   the majority of cases arise before age 20 years.

4.28   The following statements apply to alcoholic dementia.

(a)   It is more common in those who drink in bouts than those who drink continuously.

(b)   It is synonomous with Korsakov's syndrome.

(c)   It develops more readily in alcoholics over the age of 50.

(d)   Improvement usually occurs with abstinence.

(e)   Its presence can be demonstrated by CT scan in over half of alcoholic in-patients.

	Ctn	Dbt	Gu

4.29 In hyperthyroidism:

(a) women are more often affected than men.

(b) irritability is common.

(c) apathy may occur.

(d) cognitive impairment does not occur.

(e) appetite is reduced.

4.30 The following occur with increased frequency in patients with multiple sclerosis.

(a) Euphoria.

(b) Hypomania.

(c) Depression.

(d) Paranoid psychosis.

(e) Dementia.

4.31 Tardive dyskinesia:

(a) is more likely to occur in the elderly.

(b) occurs only in those treated with neuroleptics.

(c) can be produced by any drug which inhibits dopaminergic transmission.

(d) reflects dopaminergic underactivity.

(e) can be helped by anticholinergic medication.

	Ctn	Dbt	Gu

4.32 Bleuler considered the following to be primary symptoms of schizophrenia.

(a) Apophany.

(b) Autism.

(c) Affective blunting.

(d) Ambivalence.

(e) Akinesia.

4.33 The "dopamine hypothesis" of schizophrenia is supported by:

(a) the coexistence of schizophrenia and Parkinson's disease in the same individual.

(b) the model of amphetamine-induced psychosis.

(c) the therapeutic efficacy of haloperidol in schizophrenia.

(d) the homovanilic acid concentrations found in the CSF of acute schizophrenics.

(e) the serum prolactin levels found in drug-free schizophrenics.

	Ctn	Dbt	Gu

4.34 The following are considered characteristic of schizophrenic thought disorder.

(a) Prolixity.

(b) Overinclusiveness.

(c) Derailment.

(d) Loosening of associations.

(e) Clang associations.

4.35 The following tend to indicate a good prognosis in schizophrenia.

(a) Incongruity of affect.

(b) Confusion.

(c) Schizoid premorbid personality.

(d) Depressive symptoms.

(e) Echo de la pensée.

4.36 The following statements are true of schizoaffective psychosis.

(a) The prognosis is poorer than for affective psychoses.

(b) There is a raised incidence of schizophrenia in relatives.

(c) There is a raised incidence of affective psychosis in relatives.

(d) By definition, it does not recur.

(e) It is a term introduced by Magnan.

	Ctn	Dbt	Gu

4.37 **The following are consistent with a diagnosis of depressive illness.**

(a) Delusions of poverty.

(b) Delusions of reference.

(c) Delusions of sinfulness.

(d) Delusions of having been poisoned.

(e) Delusions that the patient is dead.

4.38 **The dominant X-linked gene hypothesis of the inheritance of manic-depressive illness:**

(a) was first advanced by Winokur and his colleagues.

(b) would require every daughter of manic-depressive fathers to be affected.

(c) is disproved by the fact that men and women are affected with equal frequency.

(d) is supported by the fact that father to son transmission does not occur.

(e) is supported by an association between colour blindness and manic-depressive illness in some families.

	Ctn	Dbt	Gu

4.39 **The psychological well-being of women after hysterectomy:**

(a) is usually poorer than preoperatively.

(b) is poorer than that of general population samples.

(c) is poorer when bilateral oopherectomy is also performed.

(d) correlates with the degree of organic uterine pathology.

(e) is poorer in younger women.

4.40 **The following are associated with an increased risk of suicide.**

(a) Adolescence.

(b) Divorce.

(c) Unemployment.

(d) Onset of war.

(e) Alcoholism.

	Ctn	Dbt	Gu

4.41   In depressive neurosis:

(a)   nihilistic delusions are common.   ___ ___ ___

(b)   anxiety is a common feature.   ___ ___ ___

(c)   the risk of suicide is as high as in
      psychotic depression.   ___ ___ ___

(d)   increased appetite with weight gain is
      at least as common as diminished
      appetite with weight loss.   ___ ___ ___

(e)   there is always an abnormal premorbid
      personality.   ___ ___ ___

4.42   Obsessional neurosis:

(a)   is one of the least common neurotic
      disorders.   ___ ___ ___

(b)   rarely has an acute onset.   ___ ___ ___

(c)   seldom begins after 50 years of age.   ___ ___ ___

(d)   occurs more commonly in patients of
      low intelligence.   ___ ___ ___

(e)   almost invariably has a clearly defined
      precipitant.   ___ ___ ___

	Ctn	Dbt	Gu

4.43 Depersonalization:

(a) may be accompanied by déjà vu experiences.

(b) occurs in depressive illness.

(c) may be induced by extreme fatigue.

(d) usually has a gradual onset.

(e) is usually accompanied by a loss of insight.

4.44 The following are dissociative reactions.

(a) Fugue.

(b) Trance.

(c) Hysterical amnesia.

(d) Sleeptalking (somniloquy).

(e) De Clérambault's syndrome.

4.45 Pathological gambling:

(a) is usually associated with depressive illness.

(b) carries an increased risk of parasuicide.

(c) is usually associated with a disturbed appreciation of the value of money.

(d) has good a prognosis following aversion therapy.

(e) is an obsessive - compulsive disorder.

	Ctn	Dbt	Gu

**4.46 In the acute stages of anorexia
nervosa:**

(a) patients often show non-suppression
on the DST.

(b) cortisol levels are usually lowered.

(c) there are often abnormalities in
ADH secretion.

(d) CSF noradrenaline is increased.

(e) CSF homovanilic acid is increased.

**4.47 Views on the aetiology of anorexia
nervosa are correctly paired with the
authors below.**

(a) Triangulation in covert parental
conflict: Minuchin.

(b) Primary hypothalamic dysfunction:
Russell.

(c) Atypical affective disorder: Clouston.

(d) Paralysing sense of ineffectiveness:
Bruch.

(e) Learned abnormal eating behaviour:
Crisp.

	Ctn	Dbt	Gu

4.48 Physical complications of bulimia nervosa include:

(a) menstrual irregularities.

(b) cardiac arrhythmias.

(c) erosion of dental enamel.

(d) hoarseness.

(e) parotid gland enlargement.

4.49 In psychopathic (antisocial) personality disorder:

(a) subnormal IQ is common.

(b) antisocial behaviour has usually commenced by adolescence.

(c) neurotic symptoms are rare.

(d) there is often widespread slow wave activity on the EEG.

(e) conditioned responses are quickly acquired.

	Ctn	Dbt	Gu

4.50 Insomnia is:

(a) more often reported by women than by men. ___ ___ ___

(b) uncommon among alcoholics. ___ ___ ___

(c) associated with obesity and apnoea in younger males. ___ ___ ___

(d) associated in the elderly with a compensatory rise in the proportion of slow wave sleep. ___ ___ ___

(e) less common among heavy smokers than non-smokers. ___ ___ ___

4.51 Neuroses commonly associated with psychogenic pain are:

(a) anxiety neurosis. ___ ___ ___

(b) depressive neurosis. ___ ___ ___

(c) obsessive-compulsive neurosis. ___ ___ ___

(d) hysterical neurosis. ___ ___ ___

(e) hypochondriacal neurosis. ___ ___ ___

4.52 For the following conditions the risk for females is greater than for males.

(a) Manic-depressive psychosis. ___ ___ ___

(b) Acute intermittent porphyria. ___ ___ ___

(c) Schizophrenia. ___ ___ ___

(d) Huntington's chorea. ___ ___ ___

(e) Idiopathic Parkinsonism. ___ ___ ___

	Ctn	Dbt	Gu

4.53 Transsexualism:

(a) is equally common in both sexes.

(b) is usually manifested before puberty.

(c) is usually associated with sexual
arousal during cross-dressing.

(d) is due to a chromosomal abnormality.

(e) is associated with little interest in
sexual activity.

**4.54 The following are features of
delirium tremens.**

(a) Topographical disorientation.

(b) Blunted affect.

(c) Pyrexia.

(d) Tachycardia.

(e) Dilated pupils.

	Ctn	Dbt	Gu

**4.55 The following statements are true
of disulfiram.**

(a) It inhibits the metabolism of alcohol
to acetaldehyde.

(b) It is contraindicated in patients with
ischaemic heart disease.

(c) Patients who cease to take it can
generally drink without adverse
effects 24 hours later.

(d) In combination with alcohol,
hypertension occurs.

(e) In combination with alcohol, dyspnoea
occurs.

**4.56 The following statements apply
to amphetamines.**

(a) Tolerance does not develop.

(b) They are effective in the treatment of
narcolepsy.

(c) Psychological dependence can occur.

(d) When psychosis develops it is usually
in the setting of chronic drug use.

(e) Visual hallucinations are more common
in amphetamine psychosis than in
schizophrenia.

	Ctn	Dbt	Gu

4.57 The following are recognised complications of heroin abuse.

(a) Greater than ten-fold increase in mortality rate.

(b) Alopecia.

(c) Hepatic encephalopathy.

(d) Testicular atrophy.

(e) Acute pulmonary oedema.

4.58 Shoplifting:

(a) is more common among menopausal than nonmenopausal middle-aged women.

(b) is equally common in juveniles of both sexes.

(c) commonly occurs whilst the individual is intoxicated.

(d) occurs more often among pregnant than non-pregnant women.

(e) among juveniles is likely to occur along with other deviant behaviour.

	Ctn	Dbt	Gu

4.59 To be considered fit to plead at the time of the trial the defendant must be able to:

(a) challenge a juror.

(b) examine a witness.

(c) follow the progress of the trial.

(d) instruct counsel.

(e) understand the charge.

4.60 The use of hypnosis is associated with:

(a) Bernheim.

(b) Freud.

(c) Braid.

(d) Cerletti.

(e) Elliotson.

PAPER 5

	Ctn	Dbt	Gu

5.1 Nocturnal enuresis:

(a) occurs more commonly in socially
     deprived children.   ___ ___ ___

(b) occurs only during REM sleep.   ___ ___ ___

(c) is usually helped by urethral
     dilatation.   ___ ___ ___

(d) results from urinary tract infections
     in 20-30% of cases.   ___ ___ ___

(e) occurs at least once a week in over
     1% of 9 year olds.   ___ ___ ___

5.2 Children who sustain head injuries:

(a) are more likely to be boys.   ___ ___ ___

(b) commonly have shown behavioural
     problems before the injury.   ___ ___ ___

(c) have a significantly increased likeli-
     hood of subsequent psychiatric disorder,
     irrespective of the severity of
     the injury.   ___ ___ ___

(d) may show substantial recovery for up to
     12 months.   ___ ___ ___

(e) are more likely to come from socially
     disadvantaged families.   ___ ___ ___

	Ctn	Dbt	Gu

5.3 Phobias commonly encountered in pre-school children include:

(a) insect phobias.

(b) agoraphobia.

(c) animal phobias.

(d) social phobias.

(e) height phobias.

5.4 Compared to boys, adolescent girls are more likely to:

(a) indulge in masturbation.

(b) display heterosexual interests earlier.

(c) have more sexual partners.

(d) suffer from depression.

(e) reach puberty earlier.

5.5 In Gilles de la Tourette's syndrome:

(a) males are more often affected than females.

(b) the onset is usually before 11 years of age.

(c) the tics can be inhibited by voluntary control.

(d) the tics are usually ameliorated by haloperidol.

(e) intelligence is usually subnormal.

	Ctn	Dbt	Gu

5.6 The following statements about school refusal are correct.

(a) The highest rates are in primary school children.

(b) Boys and girls are affected in equal numbers.

(c) It usually has a sudden onset in older children.

(d) School refusers usually remain at home with their parents' consent.

(e) There is rarely a specific precipitating event.

5.7 The following statements apply to Down's syndrome.

(a) The risk of an affected child is higher than 1/100 for mothers over 40 years of age.

(b) All affected children have Trisomy 21.

(c) It can be diagnosed prenatally by amniocentesis.

(d) It is the commonest diagnosable condition found in severely mentally handicapped populations.

(e) Mosaics exist who may exhibit only limited stigmata of the disease.

	Ctn	Dbt	Gu

5.8 The following are metabolic disorders associated with mental handicap.

(a) Tay-Sachs' disease.

(b) Galactosaemia.

(c) Hartnup's disease.

(d) Klinefelter's syndrome.

(e) Phenylketonuria.

5.9 Phenylketonuria:

(a) was discovered by Folling.

(b) is caused by an excess of the enzyme phenylalanine hydroxylase.

(c) results in mental handicap unless the appropriate diet is instituted within the first six months of life.

(d) must be treated with total exclusion of phenylalanine from the diet.

(e) can be detected in the urine of neonates with the Guthrie test.

| | Ctn | Dbt | Gu |

5.10 In the Lesch-Nyhan syndrome:

(a) the high levels of uric acid are
responsible for the major features.

(b) low levels of hypoxanthine phosphoribosyl
transferage (HPRT) always lead to a
clinical manifestation of the syndrome.

(c) intellectual impairment is not
always present.

(d) self-mutilation invariably
follows total absence of enzyme
activity.

(e) early treatment with allopurinol will
prevent neurological disorder and self-
mutilation.

5.11 Systematic desensitization requires:

(a) flooding.

(b) the construction of a hierarchy.

(c) response prevention.

(d) modelling.

(e) an anxiety-inhibiting response.

	Ctn	Dbt	Gu

**5.12 The following statements about
transference are correct.**

(a) Freud distinguished between positive
transference which facilitated
psychotherapy and that which impeded it. ___ ___ ___

(b) Freud believed that transference did
not readily occur in the functional
psychoses. ___ ___ ___

(c) "Acting in the transference" refers to
the therapist's tendency to act out the
patient's wishes. ___ ___ ___

(d) "Transference of defence" includes the
repetition of measures used by the
patient to protect himself against
childhood libidinal urges. ___ ___ ___

(e) According to Klein, the patient's
transference relates very largely to
experiences in the 1st year of life. ___ ___ ___

**5.13 Major developments in family therapy
have been introduced by:**

(a) Haley. ___ ___ ___

(b) Satir. ___ ___ ___

(c) Skynner. ___ ___ ___

(d) Rogers. ___ ___ ___

(e) Minuchin. ___ ___ ___

	Ctn	Dbt	Gu

5.14 Successful classical conditioning:

(a) requires the conditioned stimulus to be presented within seconds after the unconditioned stimulus.

(b) can be measured by the magnitude of the response.

(c) confirms the "Law of Effect".

(d) can be measured by the latency of the conditioned response following the conditioned stimulus.

(e) depends on "successive approximations".

5.15 An Ego-state:

(a) is a basic motivating factor of human behaviour.

(b) is a complementary transaction.

(c) is a cohesive system of thoughts and feelings.

(d) is a term coined by Jung.

(e) is usually destructive and motivated by hidden desires.

5.16 The following statements are true of cognitive therapy.

(a) Self-examination by the patient is avoided.

(b) The patient's thoughts about himself are incorrect because of faulty learning.

(c) The main priority is to promote realistic thinking.

(d) "Contingency contracting" is used to increase the likelihood of a favourable outcome.

(e) Lewin's Field Theory laid the foundations to its basic principles.

5.17 In depressive illness, the following would be considered indications for ECT.

(a) Stupor.

(b) Failure to respond to a ten day course of tricyclic antidepressants.

(c) Retardation.

(d) Paranoid delusions.

(e) Schizophreniform symptoms.

	Ctn	Dbt	Gu

5.18 In a patient undergoing ECT, the following can lower the fit threshold.

(a) Premedication with chlorpromazine.

(b) Premedication with chlordiazepoxide.

(c) The use of suxamethonium as a muscle relaxant.

(d) Isolation of the forearm with a sphygmomanometer cuff.

(e) Ventilation of the patient with pure oxygen.

5.19 The following drugs have potentially dangerous interactions with monoamine oxidase inhibitors.

(a) Pethidine.

(b) L-dopa.

(c) Methylamphetamine.

(d) Aspirin.

(e) Warfarin.

	Ctn	Dbt	Gu

5.20 Compared with amitriptyline, clomipramine:

(a) causes fewer unwanted effects.

(b) has greater effect on 5-HT reuptake.

(c) is more often used in obsessional states.

(d) has lesser sedative effect.

(e) is safer in overdose.

5.21 The symptoms of benzodiazepine withdrawal syndrome:

(a) tend to be more severe after oxazepan than after diazepam.

(b) are more likely after prolonged use.

(c) do not persist longer than 10 days.

(d) can be ameliorated by propranolol.

(e) can be ameliorated by substituting oxazepam for diazepam prior to discontinuation.

	Ctn	Dbt	Gu

5.22 Haloperidol:

(a) is a phenothiazine.

(b) is metabolised by the liver.

(c) induces production of hepatic enzymes.

(d) has a plasma half-life of 8 to 12 hours.

(e) is a more potent blocker of dopamine receptors than chlorpromazine.

5.23 Acute dystonic reactions produced by neuroleptics:

(a) rarely appear within 24 hours of starting the drug.

(b) are dose-related.

(c) should be treated with oral procyclidine.

(d) most commonly affect the elderly.

(e) include torticollis.

5.24 In late paraphrenia:

(a) the incidence is similar in both sexes.

(b) first-rank symptoms of schizophrenia are rare.

(c) over 20% of patients are deaf.

(d) patients usually develop dementia.

(e) delusions persist after treatment in the majority of cases.

	Ctn	Dbt	Gu

5.25 In Alzheimer's disease:

(a) the cerebral cortex is predominantly affected.

(b) the fronto-temporal region is usually first affected.

(c) the EEG is often normal.

(d) brain acetyl cholinesterase is increased.

(e) brain choline acetyltransferase is decreased.

5.26 When adults suffer a closed head injury:

(a) an accurate prognosis can be reached six months later.

(b) post-traumatic neurosis is the commonest psychiatric disorder.

(c) epilepsy results in over 50% of cases.

(d) intellectual function is more seriously affected by injuries to the dominant hemisphere.

(e) the likelihood of intellectual impairment rises with increasing age.

	Ctn	Dbt	Gu

5.27 The epileptic threshold is lowered by:

(a) steroids.

(b) benzodiazepines.

(c) chlorpromazine.

(d) amitriptyline.

(e) amphetamines.

5.28 The following are features of Wernicke's encephalopathy.

(a) Lateral nystagmus.

(b) Ataxia.

(c) Ptosis.

(d) Confusional state.

(e) Paralysis of conjugate gaze.

5.29 Carbon monoxide poisoning:

(a) can be followed by a latent period prior to the onset of neuropsychiatric symptoms.

(b) has become a more common method of suicide in the UK over the last 25 years.

(c) commonly induces a paranoid psychosis.

(d) often induces mild intellectual impairment.

(e) often induces Parkinsonism.

	Ctn	Dbt	Gu

5.30 In vitamin B$_{12}$ deficiency:

(a) the majority of patients have associated
cognitive impairment.

(b) the EEG is usually abnormal.

(c) mental symptoms are always apparent
when the deficiency is severe.

(d) mild dysmnesic symptoms tend to
respond to hydroxycobalamin.

(e) the deficiency can be secondary to
a dietary folate deficiency.

5.31 In acute intermittent porphyria:

(a) excessive quantities of porphobilinogen
are excreted in the urine.

(b) men are more often clinically affected
than women.

(c) affected individuals may remain
symptom free.

(d) the onset is usually in childhood.

(e) the transmission is through autosomal
recessive genes.

	Ctn	Dbt	Gu

5.32 The following are first rank symptoms of schizophrenia.

(a) Somatic passivity experiences.

(b) Thought echo.

(c) Delusional mood.

(d) Delusional memory.

(e) Delusional perception.

5.33 For schizophrenics living with "high expressed emotion" families:

(a) there is an increased relapse rate.

(b) relapse rates are higher in the unmarried.

(c) maintenance phenothiazines are of negligible benefit.

(d) criticism is usually directed at the florid features of the patient's illness.

(e) the prognosis can be improved by reducing the amount of contact between the patient and his family.

	Ctn	Dbt	Gu

5.34 **Studies of adopted children, one of whose biological parents is schizophrenic, have shown that:**

(a) these children have an increased risk of developing schizophrenia.

     ___ ___ ___

(b) these children have a lifetime risk of over 30% of developing schizophrenia.

     ___ ___ ___

(c) these children have an increased risk of developing one of the "schizophrenic spectrum disorders".

     ___ ___ ___

(d) schizophrenia can be inherited as an X-linked recessive gene.

     ___ ___ ___

(e) the later the separation from the schizophrenic parent, the greater the likelihood of the child's becoming schizophrenic.

     ___ ___ ___

5.35 **The negative symptoms of schizophrenia include:**

(a) blunting of affect.

     ___ ___ ___

(b) overactivity.

     ___ ___ ___

(c) tardive dyskinesia.

     ___ ___ ___

(d) thought disorder.

     ___ ___ ___

(e) apathy.

     ___ ___ ___

	Ctn	Dbt	Gu

5.36   In Capgras' syndrome, the patient:

(a)   believes his own identity has been
        changed.

⎯⎯ ⎯⎯ ⎯⎯

(b)   engages in "mirror gazing".

⎯⎯ ⎯⎯ ⎯⎯

(c)   almost invariably shows cognitive
        impairment.

⎯⎯ ⎯⎯ ⎯⎯

(d)   commonly has a functional psychosis.

⎯⎯ ⎯⎯ ⎯⎯

(e)   is commonly perplexed.

⎯⎯ ⎯⎯ ⎯⎯

**5.37   Compared with unipolar depression, in
            bipolar affective disorder:**

(a)   there tends to be an earlier age of
        onset.

⎯⎯ ⎯⎯ ⎯⎯

(b)   patients tend to be more neurotic
        premorbidly.

⎯⎯ ⎯⎯ ⎯⎯

(c)   episodes of illness tend to last
        longer.

⎯⎯ ⎯⎯ ⎯⎯

(d)   episodes of illness tend to recur
        more frequently.

⎯⎯ ⎯⎯ ⎯⎯

(e)   first degree relatives show higher
        rates of bipolar illness.

⎯⎯ ⎯⎯ ⎯⎯

	Ctn	Dbt	Gu

5.38 "Secondary mania" is associated with the use of the following drugs.

(a) Alcohol.

(b) Levodopa.

(c) Bromocriptine.

(d) Amphetamines.

(e) Heroin.

5.39 Puerperal psychosis:

(a) is more common in primiparous women.

(b) is less common after Caesarian section.

(c) usually begins within 24 hours of delivery.

(d) is most usually a schizophrenic psychosis.

(e) seldom responds to ECT.

5.40 Durkheim described the following types of suicide.

(a) Egoistic.

(b) Stoic.

(c) Altruistic.

(d) Anomic.

(e) Idealistic.

	Ctn	Dbt	Gu

5.41 According to George Brown and his colleagues, "vulnerability factors" to depression include:

(a) loss of father before 11 years.

(b) loss of mother before 11 years.

(c) lack of an intimate, confiding relationship.

(d) two children at home under the age of 10 years.

(e) unemployment outside the home.

5.42 According to the traditional psychoanalytic theory of the neuroses:

(a) anxiety is defined as the reaction to a real external danger.

(b) projection is the principal defence underlying phobias.

(c) repression is the same as suppression.

(d) anxiety motivates the ego to control basic drives by means of defences.

(e) castration anxiety is prominent in the male child at the Oedipal stage.

	Ctn	Dbt	Gu

5.43 In obsessional neurosis, obsessional rituals:

(a) are best treated using modelling.

(b) are not directly pleasurable for the patient.

(c) are experienced by the patient as being guided by an external force.

(d) can occur in response to auditory hallucinations.

(e) are identical to those which occur in childhood as natural phenomena.

5.44 The counterphobic attitude:

(a) was defined first by Federn.

(b) is an attempt to master fear.

(c) is the same as countertransference.

(d) may represent a denial of threat.

(e) is a form of obsessive-compulsive neurosis.

	Ctn	Dbt	Gu

5.45 The hyperventilation syndrome:

(a) may include paraesthesiae.

(b) is more common in females.

(c) is more common among pre-adolescents than young adults.

(d) may give rise to nonspecific ST and T wave alterations on the ECG.

(e) may be associated with aerophagy.

5.46 The following are physical features of anorexia nervosa.

(a) Tachycardia.

(b) Cold extremities.

(c) Leukocytosis.

(d) Absence of pubic hair.

(e) Ankle oedema.

5.47 Good prognostic indicators in anorexia nervosa include:

(a) vomiting;

(b) bingeing.

(c) early age of onset.

(d) premorbid hysterical traits.

(e) premorbid neuroticism.

	Ctn	Dbt	Gu

5.48 Obesity:

(a) is more common in women than in men.

(b) is more common in the higher
social classes.

(c) is usually the result of significant
psychiatric morbidity.

(d) is almost always the result of
substantial overeating.

(e) has no genetic basis.

5.49 In Briquet's syndrome:

(a) women are affected more often than men.

(b) there is usually an underlying
affective psychosis.

(c) somatic complaints are prominent.

(d) behavioural treatments are generally
successful.

(e) menstrual problems are common.

	Ctn	Dbt	Gu

5.50 The following statements about sleep are correct.

(a) Continued sleep loss for more than 60 hours may lead to a mild psychosis.

(b) Nightmares occur in paradoxical sleep.

(c) Tooth-grinding is an indication of a neurotic disturbance.

(d) Sleep walking is a "dissociative" state.

(e) Recent weight loss is associated with broken sleep.

5.51 Anhedonia:

(a) is a synonym for ambivalent feelings.

(b) describes an exaggerated effort to seek pleasure.

(c) is a psychoanalytic term to describe amentia.

(d) is a term introduced by Durkheim.

(e) refers to an emotional dependence on others.

	Ctn	Dbt	Gu

5.52 The following statements apply to the female menopause.

(a) It is established that there is an increased risk of psychotic depression in the perimenopausal years.   ___ ___ ___

(b) It is established that there is an increased risk of schizophrenia in the perimenopausal years.   ___ ___ ___

(c) The menopause occurs at a median age of 50 years.   ___ ___ ___

(d) Depression at the time of the menopause has been shown to be associated with severe oestrogen withdrawal symptoms.   ___ ___ ___

(e) Minor psychiatric disturbances are usually best treated with oestrogen replacement therapy.   ___ ___ ___

5.53 Lesbians are less likely than male homosexuals to:

(a) be charged with sexual molestation of children.   ___ ___ ___

(b) be promiscuous.   ___ ___ ___

(c) display a positive dislike of the opposite sex.   ___ ___ ___

(d) cohabit with a sexual partner.   ___ ___ ___

(e) want to have children.   ___ ___ ___

	Ctn	Dbt	Gu

5.54 The following are typical of alcohol withdrawal.

(a) Hypersomnia.

(b) Tremor.

(c) Bradycardia.

(d) Sweating.

(e) Nightmares.

5.55 The level of alcohol consumption per head in the UK population:

(a) has risen since the 1950's.

(b) is higher than in France.

(c) is affected by changes in the price of alcohol.

(d) is now higher in women than in men.

(e) is significantly higher in Scotland than in England.

5.56 Cocaine:

(a) has a depressant effect on the CNS.

(b) blocks the re-uptake of brain amines.

(c) induces anergia.

(d) rapidly induces physical dependence.

(e) can induce a paranoid psychosis.

	Ctn	Dbt	Gu

5.57 The Home Office should be notified about abusers of the following drugs.

(a) Barbiturates.

(b) Methadone.

(c) Heroin.

(d) Cocaine.

(e) Amphetamines.

5.58 Morbid jealousy:

(a) is more likely to occur in alcoholism than in psychotic disorders.

(b) may be the first sign of a psychotic illness.

(c) is twice as common in men as in women.

(d) is associated with overt homosexuality.

(e) is also known as "psychose passionelle".

132

		Ctn	Dbt	Gu

5.59 The following statements about arson are true.

(a) Eighty-five per cent of arsonists are male.

(b) Sexual excitement associated with arson is a poor prognostic feature.

(c) The peak incidence for males is 17 years.

(d) The peak incidence for females is 30 years.

(e) Fire setting in children is predominantly a group activity.

5.60 These are correct statements.

(a) Krafft-Ebings' work with syphilis encouraged the view that mental illness was due to physical disease.

(b) Janet's observations increased our understanding of unconscious mental processes.

(c) Bleuler showed that the features of "dementia praecox" were secondary to the group of illnesses he labelled "schizophrenia".

(d) Moniz pioneered the introduction of leucotomy.

(e) Jaspers emphasized the value of phenomenology.

PAPER 1 — ANSWERS

1.1   (a) F (b) T (c) T (d) F (e) F.

(a)   There is no association between IQ and school refusal.

(d)   The peak incidence of school refusal occurs between 11 and 13 years of age.

(e)   Even after normal school attendance has been achieved, neurotic disturbances continue in about 50% of cases.

References: Berg (1983), Hersov (1985b).

1.2   (a) F (b) F (c) F (d) F (e) T.

(a)   There is evidence that abuse is more likely among very young parents.

(b)   About one third of children do not have their injuries reported by their parents until the following morning, and another third are delayed for up to 4 days.

(c)   Although it is commonly claimed that premature babies are at greater risk of child abuse than normal babies, conclusive evidence to support this claim is lacking.

(d)   Abusing mothers show lower levels of physical and verbal interaction with their children compared to non-abusing mothers.

Reference: Mrazek and Mrazek (1985).

1.3 (a) T (b) F (c) T (d) F (e) F.

(b) Fire-setting is usually a group activity.

(c) These children show high rates of breaking and entering, stealing and truancy.

(d) Fire-setters tend to be from socially deprived backgrounds, with high levels of paternal unemployment and parental separation.

(e) As a group, fire-setters are younger than other conduct-disordered children.

Reference: Wolff (1985a).

1.4 (a) F (b) T (c) T (d) F (e) F.

Gilles de la Tourette's syndrome comprises the triad of multiple tics, involuntary utterances which are often obscene (coprolalia), and onset in childhood or adolescence. Repetition of others' speech (echolalia) and of others' actions (echopraxia) are also common.

Reference: Enoch and Trethowan (1979).

1.5 (a) F (b) T (c) T (d) T (e) F.

(a) Ratings by primary school teachers are highly predictive of subsequent delinquency.

(d) There is evidence that delinquents display autonomic under-reactivity. It is not clear whether this is due to genetic differences or to a learned adaptation to chronic environmental stress.

Reference: West (1985).

1.6 (a) T (b) T (c) T (d) F (e) T.

(c) Persistent bed-wetters are more likely to have suffered anxiety-provoking life events during their pre-school years.

(d) Most enuretic children are psychologically normal.

(e) About one third of children with urinary tract infections are enuretic.

References: Berg (1981), Wolff (1983b).

1.7 (a) T (b) T (c) T (d) F (e) F.

(d) Microcephaly is associated with this condition.

(e) This is a feature of Turner's syndrome.

Reference: Gath (1985).

1.8 (a) T (b) F (c) F (d) T (e) T.

(b) If untreated, the majority are severely handicapped, although a wide range of intellectual competence has been reported.

(c) Overactivity with stereotyped movements is commonly seen in such children.

(d) Early diagnosis is particularly important since a low phenylalanine diet results in substantial improvement, especially if initiated when the child is only a few weeks old. There are other less easily treated variants of PKU, known as malignant hyperphenylalaninaemia, depending on the specific enzyme deficiencies.

(e) This test measures the phenylalanine level in the blood using a bacteriological procedure.

Reference: Tredgold and Soddy (1970).

1.9 (a) F (b) T (c) T (d) T (e) F.

(a), (e) These are associated with early infantile autism.

1.10 (a) T (b) T (c) F (d) F (e) T.

(c) This is a metabolic disorder also called hepatolenticular degeneration. It is a disorder of copper metabolism with a recessive mode of transmission.

(d) This is an X-linked recessive condition in which there is an elevation of blood urate levels.

Reference: Syzmanski and Crocker (1985).

1.11 (a) T (b) F (c) F (d) T (e) T.

(a), (c), (d), (e) In systematic desensitization the patient learns to cope in turn with a series of anxiety-provoking stimuli while relaxed. The patient may be required to encounter these stimuli in vivo or in imagination, although the former seems to be a more effective means of relieving the patient of anxiety. Wolpe, the pioneer of this form of therapy, commonly used hypnosis as a means of inducing a state of deep relaxation.

(b) Response prevention is a method used to treat rituals. As the name suggests, the patient is deliberately prevented from carrying out ritualistic behaviours.

Reference: Walker (1982).

1.12 (a) T (b) T (c) T (d) F (e) F.

(a) This approach involves intensive therapy with various
      members of a family in different combinations.

(b) This occurs when parents cannot adapt to their childrens'
      leaving home, partly because of their own fear of being
      left alone together.

(c) Sculpting is a technique whereby the therapist asks the
      members of the family to create a physical representation
      of their family relationships by the position of their
      bodies.

(d) Jung introduced this term to refer to the psychic material
      outside the realm of awareness that is common to mankind
      in general.

(e) According to Piaget, circular reactions occur in the
      sensorimotor phase of development (0-2 years). They are
      reactions in which the completion of a response is the
      stimulus for its repetition.

Reference: Glick and Kessler (1974).

1.13 (a) F (b) T (c) T (d) T (e) F.

(a) It is psychoanalytic therapy which emphasizes the
      therapeutic value of the patient gaining insight.

(e) The behavioural approach does not require a thorough
      understanding of the original cause(s) of a disorder: it
      is more important for the behavioural therapist to
      identify the factors which are currently maintaining the
      maladaptive behaviour or symptoms.

Reference: Kazdin (1982).

1.14 (a) F (b) T (c) F (d) T (e) T.

(a) Albert Ellis developed Rational-Emotive Therapy which
     stresses problem-solving.

(b), (d), (e) E. Berne (1910 - 1970), a Freudian analyst by
     training, developed Transactional Analysis as a brief form
     of therapy which enables the patient to become aware of
     certain states of mind and the behaviour associated with
     them. The former are the so-called Ego-states of
     "Parent", "Adult" and "Child". In addition, Game Analysis
     helps the patient to recognise how he becomes involved in
     certain interpersonal transactions ("games") which prevent
     open and intimate relationships because they have hidden,
     ulterior motives.

(c) Assertive Training is a form of behaviour therapy in which
     the patient learns to assert previously inhibited
     behaviour.

Reference: Berne (1961).

1.15 (a) F (b) F (c) T (d) T (e) F.

(a) This is catharsis.

(b) This is acathexis.

(e) This is a compulsion.

1.16 (a) F (b) T (c) T (d) T (e) F.

(a) It was Anna Freud who first surveyed them systematically
     and comprehensively.

(e) Reaction formation develops in response to anal impulses.

Reference: Freud (1936).

1.17 (a) F (b) F (c) T (d) F (e) F.

All contraindications to ECT are relative. They must be balanced against the risks of a continuing depressive illness.

(a) It is not usual to give ECT in the three months after a myocardial infarction.

(b) ECT is safe throughout pregnancy.

(d) In the elderly, ECT may often be safer than tricyclic antidepressants, although it may be given at less frequent intervals in order to minimise confusion.

Reference: Freeman (1983c).

1.18 (a) F (b) T (c) T (d) F (e) T.

The symptoms arise on account of the sudden hypertension produced by pressor substances, which are normally inactivated by MAO in the gut and liver, gaining access to the systemic circulation. Other effects thus include headache, pallor, chest pains and cerebral haemorrhage which may be fatal.

References: Tyrer (1982b), Loudon (1983).

1.19 (a) T (b) T (c) T (d) F (e) T.

(c) A withdrawal syndrome may occur if the drug is stopped abruptly, and is characterised by malaise, nausea, restlessness and headache.

(d) It causes constipation.

Reference: Loudon (1983).

1.20 (a) F (b) T (c) F (d) F (e) F.

(c) Its half-life is 18-24 hours.

(d) It is distributed both intra and extracellularly, more evenly than sodium or potassium.

(e) Peak serum levels occur one half to 2 hours after ingestion.

Reference: Paykel (1982).

1.21 (a) T (b) T (c) T (d) F (e) T.

(d) No fatalities have been reported when benzodiazepines alone have been taken in overdose.

(e) An increased incidence of cleft lips and cleft palates has been reported in the babies of mothers who take benzodiazepines in the first trimester.

Reference: Tyrer (1982a).

1.22 (a) T (b) T (c) F (d) T (e) T.

These differences arise on account of chlorpromazine being a more potent antagonist of noradrenergic and cholinergic neurones than is haloperidol. Its anticholinergic properties make chlorpromazine less prone to induce Parkinsonian side-effects than is haloperidol.

Reference: Mackay (1982).

1.23 (a) T (b) T (c) F (d) F (e) F.

(c) The incidence is considerably higher at around 20%.

(d), (e) There is no specific treatment. The best management probably involves reduction of the dose of the neuroleptic and administration of a benzodiazepine.

Reference: Jenner and Marsden (1982).

1.24 (a) T (b) F (c) T (d) F (e) F.

(a), (c), (e) After the age of 65, the prevalence of senile
dementia rises at a virtually exponential rate. The
growing number of elderly people, and especially of very
elderly people, is thus resulting in a considerable
increase in prevalence in the UK.

(b) Old women are more prone to suffer from senile dementia
than are old men.

(d) It is usually assumed that the prevalence of senile
dementia does not show significant international
differences. Gurland et al (1983), however, in a
relatively large and well designed study, found roughly
twice the prevalence of dementia in community residents of
New York as compared to London.

References: Levy and Post (1982), Gurland et al (1983).

1.25 (a) T (b) F (c) T (d) T (e) F.

(b) Reflexes are increased.

(e) Prolixity, a lesser form of flight of ideas, occurs in
hypomania.

Reference: Folstein and McHugh (1983).

1.26 (a) F (b) F (c) T (d) T (e) F.

Patients with Korsakov's psychosis display both retrograde
amnesia (impaired ability to recall information acquired
before the onset of illness) and anterograde amnesia (an
impaired ability to learn new information).
Confabulation, contrary to popular belief, is not a
universal feature. Patients can repeat facts as they are
presented (i.e. immediate memory or "registration" is
unaffected), but he is unable to retain these facts for
any length of time. Patients are typically fairly
insightless with regard to their deficiencies in cognitive
functioning.

Reference: Victor (1983).

1.27 (a) F (b) F (c) F (d) T (e) F.

Epileptic automatisms occur during a state of clouding of consciousness occurring during or immediately after a seizure. The patient performs simple or complex actions without being aware of what is happening and, while there is often amnesia thereafter, partial recall of what occurs is also encountered.

Reference: Fenton (1972).

1.28 (a) T (b) T (c) F (d) F (e) F.

(c) Between the contraction of primary syphilis and the onset of neurosyphilitic symptoms an average of 11 years elapses, with a reported range of 5 to 25 years.

(d) Men are about three times as often affected as women.

(e) In most patients the EEG is abnormal, showing an excess of theta and slow wave activity.

References: Dewhurst (1969), Lishman (1978).

1.29 (a) F (b) T (c) F (d) F (e) F.

(a), (b) Lethargy, fatiguability and loss of spontaneity are typical, while elation and euphoria are uncommon.

(c) Depression in Parkinson's disease often responds well to tricyclics, possibly due to a combination of their antidepressant and anticholinergic properties.

(d), (e) Cognitive impairment is significantly more common than in control subjects, occurring in about one third of patients with Parkinson's disease. The degree of impairment is usually mild to moderate, and is unrelated to the course of the physical disability.

Reference: Mindham (1974).

1.30 (a) T (b) F (c) T (d) F (e) T.

Other drugs implicated in precipitating AIP include sulphonamides and methyldopa.

Reference: Robertson and Kennedy (1983).

1.31 (a) F (b) T (c) T (d) T (e) T.

(a)   It is inherited as a Mendelian dominant disorder.

(c)   In one third of cases psychiatric symptoms occur before the onset of the chorea.

(d)   Childhood onset occurs in 10-20% of cases; the average age of onset being between 35 and 42 years.

Reference: Trimble (1981).

1.32 (a) T (b) F (c) F (d) F (e) T.

(a)   This is a frequently reported but not universal finding. It may be due to the migration of pre-schizophrenic individuals, to the increased likelihood of non-native speakers being diagnosed schizophrenic, or to detection being more likely because immigrants tend to lack community support which might "conceal" the illness.

(b)   The correct figure is close to 1%.

(c)   The risk does not differ between the sexes.

(d)   Parents of schizophrenics have a normal social class distribution.

References: Cooper (1978), Kendell (1983a).

1.33   (a) F (b) F (c) F (d) F (e) F.

(a)   They were first described by Schneider.

(c)   They are quite common in mania.

(e)   Only some of the first rank symptoms (passivity experiences and thought alienation) can be considered to indicate breakdown of ego boundaries.

References: Mellor (1970), Abrams and Taylor (1981).

1.34   (a) T (b) F (c) F (d) T (e) T.

(b)   Catatonic symptoms often respond well to ECT.

(e)   This is a stereotyped posture whereby a catatonic patient may lie for long periods with his head a few inches off the bed.

References: Kendell (1983a), Hamilton (1985).

1.35   (a) F (b) F (c) F (d) T (e) T.

(a), (c)   Neither double-binding nor schismatic parenting has been demonstrated as having any importance in the aetiology or prognosis of schizophrenia.

(d), (e)   These are both qualities of high expressed emotion families.

References: Brown et al (1972), Vaughn and Leff (1976).

1.36 (a) F (b) T (c) T (d) T (e) F.

(a)   Cotard's syndrome usually presents in late middle life.

(d)   Nihilistic delusions comprise the central features of
      Cotard's syndrome. These are frequently related to the
      gastrointestinal tract eg "I have no stomach; my bowels
      have shrivelled up".

(e)   This is Capgras' syndrome.

Reference: Enoch and Trethowan (1979).

1.37 (a) T (b) F (c) T (d) T (e) F.

"Secondary mania" refers to manic behaviour with or
without grandiose delusions, and it can be produced by a
wide range of physical pathologies and by several
different drugs. It tends to arise when the CNS is
affected in the area of the hypothalamus, the basal
ganglia or the frontal lobe.

Reference: Cummings (1985).

1.38 (a) F (b) F (c) F (d) T (e) F.

(a)   It is probably becoming more common.

(b)   Females have about twice the lifetime risk of men.

(c)   Studies have failed to demonstrate that "involutional
      melancholia" is a distinct disease entity.

(d), (e) The majority of studies have found that depressive
      symptoms are more common in the divorced and separated,
      and in the lower social classes.

References: Boyd and Weissman (1982), Hagnell et al (1982).

1.39 (a) F (b) T (c) T (d) T (e) T.

Reference: Cox (1983).

1.40 (a) T (b) F (c) T (d) F (e) F.

(a) In the lower social classes parasuicide is seven times more common than it is among the upper classes. Suicide rates are more evenly distributed across the social classes.

(b) Depressive illness carries the highest risk of suicide; about 15% of patients with manic-depressive illness commit suicide.

(c) Males are at greater risk of suicide, while females are more likely than males to engage in parasuicide.

(d) Suicide occurs nore commonly in the spring and summer but there is no clear cut seasonal variation for parasuicide.

(e) Middle age and old age are associated with suicide; parasuicide is predominantly encountered among younger people.

Reference: Kreitman (1983).

1.41   (a) F (b) T (c) F (d) F (e) T.

(a)   This is a concept introduced by Spitz to describe apathy
and passivity seen in children separated from their
mothers: it involves three stages — protest, despair and
detachment.

(b), (e)   According to Seligman, the depressed patient believes
he cannot control those aspects of his life that relieve
suffering and bring gratification: he is in a state of
"learned helplessness".

(c)   The "double bind" is a concept considered by some (eg
Bateson) to be implicated in the aetiology of
schizophrenia.

(d)   Brown and his colleagues identified 4 such factors in
women which do not in themselves lead to depression except
in the presence of certain "provoking agents". The 4
vulnerability factors they found were: loss of mother
before the age of 11 years; having three or more children
at home under the age of 14 years; the lack of a confiding
relationship with a husband or intimate, and the lack of
employment outside the home.

Reference: Seligman (1975).

1.42 (a) F (b) F (c) F (d) F (e) T.

(a) It is distributed equally in both sexes.

(b) Obsessional neuroses are relatively uncommon, with an incidence in psychiatric populations between 0.1 and 4.6 per cent.

(c) Rarely does it begin in childhood; late adolescence and early adulthood are more commonly the periods at which it begins to develop.

(d) There is no evidence that ECT has a specific effect on obsessional symptoms.

(e) According to Freudian theory, obsessionals are concerned with conflicts associated with the anal stage of development, including aggressiveness versus submissiveness and order versus disorder.

Reference: Freeman (1983a).

1.43 (a) F (b) T (c) F (d) F (e) F.

(a) It occurs in both sexes with similar frequency.

(b) It appears to be more common in the lower socio-economic groups: this may be related to the different significance and communicative value accorded physical symptoms in different socio-economic groups.

(c) It predominates in the middle and later years.

(d) One follow-up study of nearly 150 patients over 31 months found 48% of patients to have a good outcome and 24% had a poor outcome. Factors which increased the likelihood of a good outcome were early diagnosis and the presence of anxiety or depression.

(e) Hypochondriacal neurosis has no generally agreed aetiology.

Reference: Pilowsky (1983).

1.44 (a) T (b) F (c) F (d) F (e) T.

(d) Briquet's syndrome was first described by a French physician in the 19th century. Since then the syndrome has been included in DSM – lll under the title "Somatization Disorder." It is characterized by multiple somatic complaints, often beginning in early adult life and running a life-long course. Although conversion symptoms may develop as part of the general picture they are not an essential feature of the syndrome.

(e) The explanation for this interesting finding is not known. It may have some symbolic value in psychological terms, or it may reflect interhemispheric functional differences.

Reference: Kendell (1983b).

1.45 (a) T (b) T (c) T (d) T (e) T.

Reference: Pincus (1978).

1.46 (a) F (b) F (c) T (d) T (e) F.

(a) Gull and Lasègue are usually credited with the first descriptions of anorexia nervosa, although Morton described similar cases two centuries earlier.

(b) It is at least 10 times as common in females as it is in males.

(d) Ballerinas, models, athletes and other women who have to control their shape rigorously have an increased incidence of anorexia nervosa.

(e) If there is a social class bias in the incidence of anorexia nervosa, then the upper social classes suffer from it more commonly.

Reference: Hsu (1983), Willi and Grossmann (1983).

1.47 (a) F (b) F (c) T (d) F (e) F.

(a) The outcome in males is probably similar to that in females.

(b), (d), (e) These are all unfavourable prognostic factors.

References: Steinhausen and Glanville (1983), Burns and Crisp (1984), Hall et al (1984).

1.48 (a) F (b) F (c) T (d) T (e) F.

Behaviour therapy for obesity (which comprises part of the approach of self-help groups such as "Weight Watchers") sees obesity as the result of abnormal eating behaviour. Therapy is thus aimed at modifying this behaviour by means of, for example, attempting to change eating style, and by restricting exposure to environmental food cues (stimulus control). As with other approaches to the treatment of obesity, relapse rates are high.

Reference: Wilson (1980).

1.49 (a) T (b) F (c) F (d) T (e) T.

Reference: Freeman (1983b).

1.50 (a) T (b) F (c) F (d) T (e) F.

Delusional mood is a relatively rare phenomenon in which the patient believes that something strange, but undefinable is going on around him. Specific delusions often occur thereafter to "explain" the delusional mood.

Reference: Hamilton (1985).

1.51 **(a)** T **(b)** T **(c)** F **(d)** F **(e)** T.

Type A behaviour is associated with easily aroused hostility, a sense of urgency about time and competitiveness. The Framingham Scale has been used to measure this type of behaviour, and the results show a correlation with neuroticism. Those who engage in Type A behaviour have an increased likelihood of suffering from coronary artery disease. The Recurrent Coronary Prevention Project claims that Type A behaviour can be reduced by cognitive behavioural modification.

Reference: Bass (1984).

1.52 **(a)** T **(b)** T **(c)** F **(d)** T **(e)** F.

The four essential features of this rare disorder are: approximate answers (Vorbeireden), clouding of consciousness, somatic conversion features and hallucinations; the latter may be auditory or visual.

(c) Nihilistic delusions (délire de négation)are the central symptom of Cotard's syndrome.

(e) Glossolalia is the name given to "speaking in tongues" i.e. speaking in a fabricated language or unknown tongue. This occurs in a variety of states including hysterical dissociation and schizophrenia.

Reference: Enoch and Trethowan (1979).

1.53 (a) T (b) F (c) T (d) F (e) T.

(a), (c) These are two of the four phases of the sexual
response defined by Masters and Johnson, the remaining two
being excitement and orgasm.

(b) "Marital schism" is a term coined by Lidz and his
colleagues to refer to a particular pattern of marital
relationship which they believed to be associated with the
development of schizophrenia.

(d) Reich introduced this term to describe what he thought was
a basic life force.

(e) As a means of reducing sexual anxiety, during "sensate
focus" the couple must limit their sexual activity to
touching gently and caressing each others' bodies. They
are not allowed to have sexual intercourse or experience
orgasm.

Reference: Masters and Johnson (1966).

1.54 (a) F (b) F (c) T (d) F (e) F.

(a) Alcohol is a short-acting drug and therefore only a few
hours of abstinence are necessary for withdrawal symptoms
to occur. Thus, they are usually experienced on wakening.

(b) Rarely withdrawal symptoms, such as hallucinations, can
occur in alcoholics who have decreased their blood alcohol
levels by moderating but not stopping their drinking.

(d) Withdrawal symptoms represent the opposite of the effects
produced by the drug ("rebound phenomena"). Since alcohol
is a sedative, withdrawal is characterised by
hyperarousal.

Reference: Victor (1983).

1.55 (a) F (b) F (c) F (d) F (e) T.

No specific features of therapy have been established as
having a beneficial effect in the treatment of alcoholism.
Patient characteristics, notably social and marital
stability, are better predictors of outcome.

Reference: Ritson and Chick (1983).

1.56 (a) T (b) T (c) F (d) F (e) T.

Reference: Ghodse (1983).

1.57 (a) T (b) T (c) F (d) T (e) F.

(c) Solvent abuse is usually a group activity.

(d) Most young people who abuse solvents do so for only a
short time and on only a few occasions.

(e) Physical dependence, if it occurs at all, is very rare.

Reference: Sourindrhin (1985).

1.58 (a) T (b) F (c) T (d) T (e) F.

A patient may be considered to have testamentary capacity
even if he is suffering from a mental illness and is
deluded, provided the disorder or delusions are considered
unlikely to influence his judgements and feelings relevant
to the provision of a will.

1.59 **(a) F (b) F (c) F (d) F (e) T.**

(a) The McNaughten Rules have never been incorporated into Scots law.

(b) They are predominantly extraverted mesomorphs.

(c) The role of the XYY karyotype in determining criminal behaviour has been exaggerated: its clinical and criminological significance remains unclear.

(d) The mentally ill are less likely to be reconvicted.

(e) It is not known why this should be so. It may reflect, for example, a specific link between cerebral dysfunction and certain crimes, such as those of violence, or it may be a secondary consequence of the patient's inability to adapt to what he sees as the stigma and disadvantages associated with epilepsy.

References: Gibbens and Robertson (1983), Macrae (1983).

1.60 **(a) T (b) F (c) T (d) F (e) T.**

(b) Cade is known for his use of lithium salts with severely disturbed manic patients. Cerletti and Bini in 1938 introduced electro-convulsive therapy as a safer and more effective method of inducing fits than camphor oil or cardiazol, the methods recommended by Meduna some years previously.

(d) Sakel was the first to use injections of insulin as a means of inducing a hypoglycaemic coma: a treatment he proposed for schizophrenia. Moreno pioneered the use of psychodrama with psychiatric patients.

PAPER 2 - ANSWERS

2.1 (a) F (b) F (c) F (d) T (e) F.

(a) Boys outnumber girls by more than 3 to 1.

(b) Retarded readers tend to have a lower verbal than performance IQ, in keeping with the strong association of speech and language delay with retarded reading.

(c) Reading retardation is associated with difficulties in telling left from right, but there is no excess of left-handed children among retarded readers.

Reference: Yule and Rutter (1985).

2.2 (a) F (b) T (c) T (d) T (e) F.

(a) It is more common in boys, although diurnal enuresis is more common among girls.

(e) No single pattern of toilet training has been established as a cause of enuresis.

References: Taylor (1983), Wolff (1983b).

2.3 (a) F (b) T (c) T (d) T (e) F.

(a) In general population surveys of adolescents, anxiety
     states and depression are the most common psychiatric
     disorders: circumscribed phobias are rare.

(e) In adolescence there is a considerable increase in the
     incidence of depressive disorders, particularly among
     females. Before puberty there is a preponderance of males
     suffering from depression but after puberty females
     predominate. To some extent this may be a consequence of
     male depressive disorders being masked by antisocial
     behaviour.

Reference: Graham and Rutter (1985).

2.4 (a) T (b) T (c) T (d) F (e) F.

Reference: International Classification of Diseases, 9th
            revision (1978).

2.5 (a) T (b) F (c) T (d) F (e) F.

(c) Indiscriminate friendliness is not a common feature of
     children taken into institutional care in later childhood.

(d), (e) Conduct disorders are associated with large families
          and marital discord.

Reference: Rutter and Gould (1985).

2.6 (a) F (b) T (c) F (d) T (e) F.

(c) It is unrelated to handedness.

(e) The age of onset is usually before 8 years of age.

Reference: Corbett (1983).

2.7 (a) F (b) T (c) T (d) T (e) T.

References: Wing (1982), Zealley (1983).

2.8 (a) T (b) T (c) F (d) T (e) F.

(a) These may include atrophy of the testes and hypospadias.

(b) This is a characteristic feature, attributable to excessive leg length in relation to the trunk.

(c) A wide range of intellectual ability has been described in Klinefelter's but mild retardation is most likely; the primary feature of which is language impairment.

(d) These patients show a considerably increased risk of psychiatric morbidity, particularly with respect to the development of depressive and paranoid symptoms.

(e) Patients with this condition are more likely to be timid and withdrawn.

Reference: Gath (1985).

2.9 (a) T (b) T (c) T (d) F (e) T.

(a) Non-dysjunction leading to trisomy 21 is strongly associated with increasing maternal age. Risks rise from 1 in 1,500 for mothers of 24 years or less to 1 in 25 for mothers of 45 years or over. Paternal age has little effect on incidence, except possibly in the case of fathers over 50 years of age.

(d) Autism is rare in Down's syndrome.

Reference: Gath (1985).

2.10 (a) T (b) F (c) T (d) F (e) T.

(b)   The IQ distribution in Turner's syndrome is virtually
       normal.

(d)   Only about 10% of children with neurofibromatosis are
       mentally subnormal, and the subnormality tends to be mild.

2.11 (a) F (b) T (c) F (d) T (e) F.

(a), (e) These are specific techniques of logotherapy devised
          by Frankl. By paradoxical intention the patient may be
          encouraged to exaggerate his symptoms rather than to fight
          them. Through dereflection the patient is enabled to
          ignore his symptoms and focus on potentially fulfilling
          aspects of life.

(b), (c), (d) Rogerian therapy emphasizes the innate potential
          of each individual for change and development. Man is
          seen as basically rational and socialized, in contrast to
          the views offered by traditional Freudian theory.
          Genuineness, empathy and unconditional positive regard are
          qualities of the therapist which are held to be necessary
          and sufficient conditions for successful therapeutic
          outcome.

References: Rogers (1951), Frankl (1968).

2.12 (a) F (b) T (c) T (d) T (e) F.

(a)   Covert sensitization involves the patient imagining scenes
       that are rewarding or punishing for emitting adaptive and
       maladaptive responses respectively.

(e)   The facilitation of insight is one of the principal aims
       of psychoanalytic therapy.

Reference: Bandura (1969).

2.13 (a) T (b) F (c) F (d) F (e) T.

(a) The "shadow" represents the unacceptable aspects of ourselves.

(b) The "action self" is Rado's term for the Ego.

(c) The individual's unique style of adapting to his social milieu is his "life-style", according to Adler.

(d) Reich coined the term "orgone" to refer to a form of energy.

(e) According to Jungian psychology, the "anima" in the case of males is the female aspect of the self; "animus" is the male aspect in females. Both are archetypal representations of predispositions or potential.

Reference: Storr (1973).

2.14 (a) T (b) T (c) F (d) F (e) T.

According to Alexander, psychoanalytic therapy helps the patient to expose himself in the therapeutic relationship to emotional situations with which he could not cope in the past. This method of therapy requires the therapist, using his understanding of the origin of the patient's problems, to recreate these situations in order that he can reality-test his fears and expectations. In the context of the therapeutic relationship he can learn to cope better with conflictual situations and relationships. Whilst therapy may facilitate this learning, it is possible for a "corrective emotional experience" to occur in the patient's daily life.

Reference: Alexander (1980).

2.15 (a) F (b) T (c) T (d) F (e) T.

Token economies employ the principles of operant conditioning, whereby desired behaviour is reinforced by tokens which can be exchanged for a variety of privileges. This system, used in many institutions, owes much to the pioneering work Ayllon and Azrin. Maxwell Jones is associated with "therapeutic communities."

Reference: Ayllon and Azrin (1968).

2.16 (a) F (b) T (c) T (d) F (e) F.

(a) Perls was responsible for the introduction of Gestalt therapy: Janov devised Primal therapy.

(b), (c), (d) Underlying Primal therapy is the principle that insight into and talking about deeply buried, painful childhood experiences is not sufficient for therapeutic change. To be relieved from his neurotic symptoms the patient must recapture specific childhood memories and act out Primals; the concentrated expression of deep infantile pain, due to the child's awareness that his parents did not love him (the Primal Trauma).

(e) The Primary Mental Abilities are those abilities which some investigators have claimed to have identified by factor analysis as the basic components of intelligence.

Reference: Janov (1970).

2.17 (a) F (b) F (c) T (d) T (e) F.

Reference: Freeman (1983c).

2.18 (a) F (b) F (c) T (d) F (e) F.

(a) Absorption of diazepam and chlordiazepoxide is surprisingly slow after IM injection. Lorazepam gives a much faster effect.

(b) Diazepam, and its metabolites, have a half-life of over 30 hours.

(e) Plasma levels are actually lower in the elderly. Their greater sensitivity to benzodiazepines is likely to arise due to the "ageing brain".

Reference: Tyrer (1982a).

2.19 (a) F (b) T (c) F (d) F (e) T.

(a) Mianserin is a tetracyclic antidepressant.

(c) The majority of trials comparing the antidepressant potency of amitriptyline and mianserin have not detected a difference between them.

(d) Mianserin does not produce ECG changes in therapeutic doses.

Reference: Barnes and Bridges (1982).

2.20 (a) T (b) T (c) T (d) F (e) F.

(a), (b) Tricyclics are particularly prone to induce serious dysrhythmias under these circumstances.

(c) Tricyclics can precipitate a typical MAOI overdose syndrome when given in combination with MAOI's, especially tranylcypromine.

(e) Tricyclics may be specifically helpful in Irritable Bowel syndrome. It is not clear whether this effect is mediated through their antidepressant or their anticholinergic properties.

References: Ford et al (1982), Loudon (1983), Orme (1984).

2.21   (a) T (b) T (c) T (d) T (e) F.

(c)   Although often given in combination with MAOI's,
      L-tryptophan can precipitate an MAOI overdose syndrome,
      especially when given in doses of 3 grams or more per day.

(e)   It has mild sedative properties.   Indeed, while unwanted
      effects are uncommon, drowsiness and nausea are the
      commonest side effects encountered.

References: Tyrer (1982b), Loudon (1983).

2.22   (a) T (b) F (c) T (d) T (e) F.

(b)   Pimozide is one of the diphenylbutylpiperidines.

(c), (d)   Pimozide is a more selective blocker of dopaminergic
      receptors than is chlorpromazine.

Reference: Mackay (1982).

2.23   a) F (b) F (c) F (d) F (e) F.

(a)   Akathisia usually appears later than acute dystonic
      reactions, but before Parkinsonian side-effects.

(b)   It occurs more commonly in women.

(d)   Alleviation of akathisia by anticholinergics is uncommon.

(e)   There is no known association with age.

References: Jenner and Marsden (1982), Mackay (1982).

2.24   (a) T (b) T (c) F (d) F (e) F.

(c)   Classically, the premorbid personalities of patients who
develop late paraphrenia show schizoid and paranoid
traits, resulting in their being isolated and eccentric.
These traits often become more extreme in the years prior
to the development of overt psychotic symptoms.

(d)   About half of such patients show depressive features.

(e)   Neuroleptic medication is the treatment of choice.

References: Grahame (1982), Post (1982).

2.25   (a) T (b) T (c) F (d) T (e) T.

(c)   SDAT tends to develop later than multi-infarct dementia.

References: Levy and Post (1982), Perry and Perry (1982).

2.26   (a) F (b) T (c) T (d) T (e) F.

(a)   In closed head injuries, the duration of post-traumatic
amnesia is a fairly reliable guide to the likelihood of
intellectual impairment. In penetrating injuries,
however, the degree of damage is less accurately reflected
by the duration of amnesia.

(c)   Injuries to the dominant hemisphere - the left hemisphere
in right handed people - is more likely to result in
intellectual impairment.

Reference: Lishman (1973).

2.27 (a) F (b) F (c) F (d) T (e) F.

(a), (e) Creutzfeld – Jakob disease (CJD) probably results
from infection with a "slow virus". It can be transmitted
from human to human (e.g. by corneal transplant), and from
human to chimpanzee by intracerebral inoculation of
affected cortical tissue.

(b), (c), (d) The central feature of CJD is intellectual
deterioration of relatively sudden onset. It tends to
have a rapidly progressive course, the majority of
patients dying within a year.

Reference: Robertson and Kennedy (1983).

2.28 (a) T (b) T (c) T (d) T (e) T.

Reference: Lishman (1978).

2.29 (a) T (b) T (c) F (d) F (e) T.

(c) The onset of psychiatric illness in hypothyroidism is
sometimes acute.

(d) Slowness of thought, memory impairment and poor
concentration are common.

Reference: Lishman (1978).

2.30 (a) T (b) F (c) T (d) F (e) F.

(a)   Over 80% do so.

(b)   Lesions predominantly affect the grey matter.

(d)   Intravenous thiamine, in a dose of 50mg, should be given immediately.

(e)   Ophthalmoplegias tend to be the earliest symptoms to recover, often doing so within a few days, while nystagmus commonly persists. Ataxia and neuropathies may persist in an attenuated form for many years.

Reference: Robertson and Kennedy (1983).

2.31 (a) F (b) F (c) T (d) T (e) F.

(a)   Tardive dyskinesia usually appears after at least 2 years continuous treatment with neuroleptics.

(b)   It disappears during sleep.

Reference: Mackay (1982).

2.32 (a) T (b) T (c) T (d) F (e) T.

References: Vaillant (1964), Stephens et al (1966).

2.33 (a) F (b) F (c) T (d) T (e) F.

The 'drift hypothesis' refers to the propensity of schizophrenics to drift down the social scale, and their resultant tendency to become concentrated in the poorer, central areas of large cities.

References: Cooper (1978), Kendell (1983a).

2.34   (a) F (b) T (c) F (d) F (e) T.

(a)   Circumstantiality involves the patient's providing a lot
      of unnecessary and trivial detail.

(d)   In perseveration of thinking ideas persist beyond the
      point at which they are relevant.   Its presence is very
      suggestive of an organic brain syndrome.

(e)   Asyndesis refers to a lack of adequate connections between
      successive thoughts.

Reference: Hamilton (1985).

2.35   (a) F (b) F (c) F (d) F (e) F.

Reference: Wing (1982b).

2.36   (a) T (b) T (c) F (d) F (e) F.

(d), (e) Both of these factors would tend to make it less
      likely that his children would develop a psychotic
      illness.

Reference: Kay (1978).

2.37   (a) T (b) T (c) F (d) T (e) F.

(d)   Persecutory delusions and delusions of reference are at
      least as common in psychotic depression as many of the
      "classical" types of depressive delusions.

(e)   Delusions of passivity are first rank symptoms of
      schizophrenia.

2.38 (a) F (b) F (c) F (d) F (e) T.

(a), (b), (c) Depressive illness causes a slight decrease in extraversion scores and a fairly large increase in neuroticism.

These changes in "personality traits" with depressive illness illustrate the pitfalls of making a diagnosis of personality disorder while a patient is psychiatrically ill.

Reference: Coppen and Metcalfe (1965).

2.39 (a) F (b) T (c) F (d) T (e) T.

After a stillbirth or perinatal death, the mother (and often the father) undergoes a grief reaction. This grieving is made more difficult by the fact that the loss is not as "concrete" as it usually is after a bereavement. It is thus helpful, (by making the loss more "concrete"), to encourage the mother to hold the dead baby and to keep photographs and other mementos. A further pregnancy should be avoided until mourning is completed, or feelings for the dead baby may be displaced on to the next baby – the "replacement child syndrome".

Reference: Bourne and Lewis (1984).

2.40 (a) T (b) F (c) F (d) F (e) F.

(b) Suicide occurs more commonly in spring and summer.

(c) Urban populations have higher rates.

(d) Although it is often alleged that there is this inverse relationship, there is no sound empirical support for this or any other relationship between suicide and homicide.

(c) Male depressives carry a higher risk.

References: Kreitman (1983), McClure (1984).

2.41 **(a)** T **(b)** T **(c)** T **(d)** T **(e)** T.

Reference: Parkes (1985).

2.42 **(a)** F **(b)** F **(c)** F **(d)** F **(e)** F.

(a) At least three quarters of sufferers are female.

(b) It is not generally associated with marital problems, but the coexistence of agoraphobia and marital problems may make treatment more difficult.

(c) Although little is known about the ultimate outcome of untreated agoraphobia, it resolves spontaneously less quickly than anxiety states.

(d) The age of onset is usually between 18 and 35 years of age.

(e) Despite its etymology, a fear of open spaces is not the major feature of agoraphobia: a fear of being away from "safe" persons or "safe" places is paramount. Usually there is a high level of generalized anxiety.

Reference: Gelder (1983).

2.43 **(a)** T **(b)** F **(c)** T **(d)** F **(e)** F.

An obsession is an intrusive and repetitive thought or image which is unacceptable and usually distressing to the patient. The content often involves dirt, aggression, orderliness and sex, but there is no association between content and prognosis. Obsessions are closely linked with compulsions which are stereotyped acts.

Reference: Rachman (1982).

2.44 (a) F (b) F (c) T (d) T (e) F.

(a)   Omnipotence of thought is "magical thinking" which occurs
      in obsessive – compulsive neuroses. It reflects the
      individual's belief that merely thinking about an event is
      enough to ensure its realization. For example, the
      patient may fear that by merely thinking about the death
      of somebody he may bring it about.

(b)   Repression is the principal defence in hysteria. It is
      the process whereby unacceptable material is rendered
      unconscious.

(e)   Primary gain occurs when the underlying conflict is
      resolved by the formation of an hysterical symptom.
      Secondary gain occurs when the symptom becomes, for
      example, the object of sympathy and attention.

Reference: Kendell (1983b).

2.45 (a) T (b) F (c) F (d) F (e) T.

      Compensation neuroses are those psychological reactions
      thought to be produced or maintained by the prospect of
      compensation. Problems of definition and methodology make
      it hard to be precise about their incidence, but they
      appear to be twice as common among working men as working
      women and more common among the less skilled and poorly
      educated. They are not related to age or to any
      particular degree of injury. There is some evidence,
      however, to suggest that the emotional reaction may be
      related to the symbolic significance of the part of the
      body injured. There is no consistent research evidence to
      confirm that these neuroses remit once compensation has
      been obtained. Collusive support from families and
      spouses appears to prolong the symptoms.

References: Weighill (1983), Tarsh and Royston (1985).

2.46 (a) F (b) F (c) F (d) T (e) T.

(a)   In about 10-15% of cases, amenorrhoea precedes significant
      weight loss.

(c)   Decreased libido is virtually invariable and, indeed, many
      cite it as a diagnostic criterion in male patients.

Reference: Russell (1970).

2.47 (a) T (b) T (c) T (d) T (e) F.

(a), (b)   Concordance for monozygotic twins is about 50%,
           compared with about 10% in dizygotic twins and siblings.

(c), (d)   This evidence can be viewed as lending support to
           including anorexia nervosa among the "depressive spectrum
           disorders".

References: Fairburn (1983a), Hudson et al (1983), Holland et
             al (1984).

2.48 (a) F (b) F (c) T (d) F (e) T.

The response of bulimia to antidepressants lends support
to the theory that it represents an atypical affective
disorder, although many would consider mood changes to be
the result, rather than the cause, of bulimia nervosa.

References: Pope et al (1983), Walsh et al (1984).

2.49 **(a) T (b) F (c) T (d) F (e) T.**

(a), (c)   The disorder was first described in 1951 by Asher,
but it has also been described by Barker as the "Hospital
Addiction Syndrome", which he thought was a more accurate
reflection of the nature of this relatively rare
condition.

(b)   The aetiology is unknown, and patients suffering from this
condition do not appear to be suffering from any clearcut
psychiatric disorder.

(d)   Patients who suffer from dysmorphophobia complain about
some presumed blemish or defect in their physical
appearance. Although their appearance may be quite normal
these patients believe their blemish or defect is obvious
to others.

Reference: Snaith (1981).

2.50 **(a) T (b) T (c) T (d) F (e) F.**

This syndrome was originally described by Gelineau in the
19th Century. The onset may be at any age. It is
characterized by day-time attacks of irresistible sleep,
sleep paralysis, cataplexy and hypnagogic
"hallucinations". The latter are probably due to the fact
that these patients pass directly into paradoxical sleep
which is associated with vivid dreams. Normal individuals
pass into orthodox sleep first.

Reference: Oswald (1983).

2.51 **(a) T (b) T (c) F (d) T (e) T.**

Autoscopy refers to the experience in which a patient
"sees himself" and knows that it is himself. It can occur
in normal people, for example, when they are exhausted or
emotionally disturbed. It occurs most commonly in
epilepsy and other organic conditions, expecially when the
parieto-occipital region of the brain is affected.

Reference: Hamilton (1985).

2.52 (a) F (b) F (c) F (d) T (e) T.

(a), (b), (c) Admission rates are falling for schizophrenia
and depressive illnesses, possibly due to the trend
towards community care.

(d) Female admission rates for alcoholism are rising, while
male rates are stabilising, indicating that the gap
between female and male rates for alcohol-related problems
is narrowing.

2.53 (a) T (b) F (c) F (d) F (e) T.

(c) Kinsey and his colleagues included particular samples (eg
prisoners) which may have inflated their prevalence rates.

(b) It should be noted that many homosexuals are well-adapted
and content, but overall they show a higher rate of
psychological problems than do heterosexual controls.
Some of this may be due to the social stigma they
experience.

(c) In prisons and other similar settings violent homosexual
activity may occur, probably as a means of asserting
social dominance. In society, however, homosexual
assaults in homosexual settings are uncommon.

(e) There is some evidence that homosexual tendencies may be
potentiated by the failure of sex differentiation of the
brain due to abnormal hormonal levels during critical
stages of foetal development.

References: Bancroft (1983), West (1983).

2.54 (a) F (b) T (c) F (d) F (e) T.

(a)   Drinking problems, usually undetected, are very common in
      medical inpatients. Jarman and Kellett (1979) found 20%
      of a London sample (9% of women, 29% of men) to have a
      significant alcohol-related problem.

(c)   Alcohol problems occur most commonly in the upper and
      lower social classes.

References: Mellor (1975), Jarman and Kellett (1979).

2.55 (a) T (b) F (c) F (d) F (e) T.

(a)   The mortality rate is about 10-15%.

(b)   Delirium tremens is a relatively rare condition, occurring
      in less than 5% of alcoholic admissions.

(c)   The majority of patients are symptomatic for less than 3
      days.

(d)   A well lit room is to be preferred, thus minimising
      ambiguities which can exacerbate confusion, as in any
      delirious condition.

References: Ritson and Chick (1983), Victor (1983).

2.56 (a) T (b) T (c) T (d) F (e) F.

(a), (b), (c) Acute psychotic reactions to cannabis usually
      last for a few hours and, in addition to paranoid
      delusions and visual and auditory hallucinations,
      confusion and disorientation occur.

Reference: Ghodse (1983).

2.57 (a) T (b) T (d) T (e) T.

Other opiate withdrawal symptoms are anxiety, yawning, mydriasis, nausea, anorexia and increased respiratory rate.

Reference: Ghodse (1983).

2.58 (a) F (b) T (c) T (d) F (e) T.

(a) A legal criterion of the definition is that sexual intercourse must have taken place.

(b) Although rarely reported by males, about 4 per cent of women reported an incestuous approach by a near relative (Bluglass, 1979).

(c) Sibling relationships are probably the most common form of incest but father-daughter cases of incest are more commonly brought to the attention of the authorities.

(d) Incest occurs in all socio-economic groups, but it is likely that incest may be detected more commonly among socially disadvantaged groups who have more contact with various legal, social and medical agencies.

Reference: Bluglass (1979).

2.59 (a) T (b) F (c) F (d) F (e) F.

(b) The majority of offenders commit this offence only once.

(c) Some violent sexual offenders do have a history of exhibitionism but the latter rarely leads on to violent sexual offences or interference with children.

(d) "Scopophilia" is a synonym for voyeurism. "Indecent exposure" is the legal offence with which those who exhibit are charged.

(e) Exhibitionism occurs throughout the range of intelligence.

Reference: Rooth (1971).

2.60 (a) F (b) T (c) T (d) T (e) F.

(a) Sprenger was co-author with Kramer of the "Malleus
     Maleficarum" (the Witches' Hammer), published in the 15th
     Century which led to the persecution, torture and death of
     "witches" many of whom would now be considered to be
     mentally disturbed individuals.

(e) Willis, the great anatomist of the 17th Century,
     emphasized the value of restraint, physical punishment and
     intimidation as means of dealing with the mentally
     disturbed.

Reference: Zilboorg (1967).

PAPER 3 - ANSWERS

3.1 (a) T (b) T (c) T (d) F (e) F.

(b) Faecal soiling is about three times commoner in boys than in girls.

(e) It is usual to consider 4 years as the age after which failure to maintain bowel control is abnormal.

Reference: Hersov (1985c).

3.2 (a) F (b) T (c) T (d) T (e) T.

(a), (b) "NOFT" refers to those children whose weight falls below the 3rd percentile but where no organic aetiology can be found. Height is also usually below the 3rd percentile, but head circumference is often normal.

(c) It is widely accepted that maladaptive parent-child interactions interfere with the child's growth and feeding.

(d) Behavioural observations confirm that NOFT children prefer less intimate social relationships, and choose to play with inanimate toys, whereas medically sick children, for whom there is an organic cause for their low weight, enjoy close personal interactions involving holding and touching.

(e) Several studies have indicated a poor prognosis for NOFT children, including reading delay, emotional and conduct disorders, and subsequent abuse by the parents.

Reference: Mrazek and Mrazek (1985).

3.3 **(a) F (b) F (c) F (d) F (e) T.**

(c) While genetic factors appear to play a part in the aetiology of Gilles de la Tourette's syndrome, the mode of transmission is not known.

(d) Although EEG abnormalities occur in about two thirds of these children, the abnormalities are non-specific and similar to those associated with other behaviour disorders.

Reference: Corbett and Turpin (1985).

3.4 **(a) F (b) T (c) T (d) F (e) T.**

(a), (b) As in adults, this disorder is becoming less common in children, but is more common in girls than in boys.

(c) Episodes of mass hysteria are good examples of the effect of identification.

(d), (e) It is rarely accompanied by conduct disorder but, in contrast with adults, it is usually accompanied by anxiety.

Reference: Wolff (1983b).

3.5 **(a) T (b) T (c) T (d) F (e) T.**

(a), (d), (e) Early language and developmental delay are likely to be associated with a poor prognosis, especially in boys who generally have a worse prognosis than girls. Especially in boys, persistent preschool problems are likely to develop into conduct disorders in later years.

Reference: Richman (1985).

3.6 (a) F (b) F (c) F (d) F (e) F.

(a), (b), (c), (d) Boys and girls are equally affected and
there is no association with class, broken homes or family
size.

(e) In general, school refusal occurs in about 5% of
psychiatrically disturbed children, although the
association is higher among adolescents than among
children at primary school.

Reference: Berg (1983).

3.7 (a) T (b) F (c) T (d) F (e) F.

In the early 1960's, Renpenning and his colleagues
reported this apparently X-linked cause of mental handicap
which is usually associated with large ears, prognathism,
macro-orchidism and serious speech impairment. It can
however occur in males who are otherwise normal.
It has been estimated to occur in about 9 per 10,000 of
the general population and in 10%-20% of mentally
handicapped males.
Prenatal identification is now feasible and there have
been claims that the Fragile X-syndrome might be remedied
by the use of folic acid.

Reference: Zealley (1983).

3.8 (a) F (b) F (c) T (d) F (e) F.

(a), (b) Tay-Sachs' disease and phenylketonuria are inherited
as autosomal recessive genes.

(d), (e) Tuberous sclerosis and neurofibromatosis are inherited
as autosomal dominant genes.

Reference: Murray and McGuffin (1983).

3.9 (a) F (b) T (c) F (d) F (e) F.

(a) These have been a popular choice of treatment, but their value has been questioned, particularly since there may be hazards associated with their longterm use, for example, loss of appetite and retarded growth.

(c) It is more common among the severely retarded.

(e) It is rarely due to manic-depressive psychosis: usually it appears to be related to structural brain abnormalities.

Reference: Reid (1982).

3.10 (a) T (b) T (c) F (d) T (e) T.

(a), (b), (d), (e) These are the 4 principal features of the Lesch-Nyhan syndrome.

Reference: Russell (1985).

3.11 (a) F (b) F (c) T (d) T (e) F.

(a) Response prevention, used mainly for treating compulsive rituals, involves the patient having to resist maladaptive behaviours for sustained periods.

(d) Response cost involves the contingent withdrawal of a reward; this is, therefore, basically a punishment.

(e) In flooding, patients are required to encounter stimuli for sustained periods at high levels of anxiety until these stimuli no longer have unwanted effects.

Reference: Rimm and Masters (1979).

3.12   (a) F (b) F (c) F (d) F (e) F.

(a)   The "manifest content" is what is reported by the patient
and represents a disguised version of the "latent
content", which reflects the hidden or unconscious meaning
of the dream.

(b)   "Secondary process" thinking is characteristic of
conscious mental activity; the latent content of dreams is
associated with "primary processes", which are
characterised by illogical and disorganised thinking.

(c)   The "Ego-ideal" is the positive aspect of the Superego,
reflecting the precepts we may try to follow.

(d)   "Dream work" refers to the mental mechanisms used by the
patient to <u>distort</u> the latent content of the dream.

(e)   Puberty marks a resurgence of the sexual drive; the
"latency period" is the period from 5 years to 12 years
during which it is claimed that there is a lack of
interest in sexual matters.

3.13   (a) T (b) T (c) F (d) T (e) F.

Frederick Perls (1893 - 1970) was a psychoanalyst who
developed Gestalt therapy. This form of therapy
emphasizes the "here and now" rather than the historical
analysis of the patient's interpersonal problems.
Patients are considered to have potential for change and,
therefore, can be expected to take a major responsibility
for their own development. The therapist plays an active
part, prescribing various activities for the patient
rather than making extensive use of interpretation as he
would in psychodynamic therapy.

Reference: Tillett (1984).

3.14 (a) T (b) T (c) F (d) F (e) T.

Reality-testing is a fundamental capacity of the Ego which helps the individual gain an objective evaluation of the world. It begins developing in childhood in accordance with the Reality Principle, which represents the demands of the external world and which modifies the demands of the competing Pleasure Principle. The latter is a psychoanalytic notion which states that an individual seeks to gain pleasure and avoid pain. Reality-testing may become impaired at times of stress or when the individual regresses. A substantial impairment of reality-testing may indicate serious mental illness.

3.15 (a) F (b) T (c) T (d) T (e) F.

(a) Kübler-Ross is known for her work with dying patients, their needs and reactions, but she has not specifically contributed to Crisis Theory.

(b) Bannister, in conjunction with Fransella, developed the Grid Test of schizophrenia.

Reference: Hobbs (1984).

3.16 (a) F (b) T (c) T (d) T (e) F.

Wolpe pioneered the technique now known as systematic desensitization. Stampfl and Levis introduced implosive techniques, the aim of which is to relieve the patient's anxiety which causes him to avoid certain situations and behaviour. Typically, the patient is required to imagine anxiety-provoking items in order that he can experience anxiety without any aversive consequences. Once he has learned that such consequences will not occur the anxiety will dissipate.

Reference: Stampfl and Levis (1967).

3.17 (a) T (b) T (c) F (d) F (e) F.

Reference: Freeman (1983c).

3.18 (a) T (b) T (c) F (d) T (e) F.

(a)   It can take over three months for the EEG to normalise after ECT.

(b)   The rise in serum prolactin which occurs within minutes of an epileptic fit can be employed to distinguish hysterical fits from genuine ones.

(c)   Plasma cortisol rises and stays high for 2 to 4 hours.

(e)   Cerebral blood flow increases considerably.

Reference: Freeman (1983c).

3.19 (a) F (b) T (c) T (d) F (e) F.

(d)   Broad bean pods must be avoided by patients on MAOI's, but this is on account of their high dopamine content.

(e)   Unlike most other cheeses, the tyramine content of cottage cheese is very low, and it is safe with MAOI's.

Reference: Tyrer (1982b).

3.20 (a) T (b) T (c) T (d) T (e) T.

Reference: Orme (1984).

3.21 (a) F (b) T (c) F (d) T (e) T.

(a), (b) While toxicity usually appears at blood levels above 1.3 mmol/l, susceptible individuals (such as the elderly) may develop symptoms at much lower plasma concentrations.

(c)   Diarrhoea is an early symptom of lithium toxicity.

(e)   While polyuria is a common side-effect of longterm lithium therapy, when lithium toxicity develops urinary output can fall due to a direct toxic effect on the kidney.

Reference: Tyrer and Shaw (1982).

3.22 (a) T (b) F (c) F (d) T (e) T.

(b), (c)   Its plasma half-life is about 27 hours, and
psychomotor impairment endures for up to 18 hours after
ingestion.   This makes it quite unsuitable as a hypnotic.

(d)   Clobazam has less effect on psychomotor performance than
equivalent doses of other benzodiazepines, with apparently
similar anxiolytic properties.

Reference: Tyrer (1982a).

3.23 (a) T (b) T (c) F (d) T (e) T.

Reference: Mackay (1982).

3.24 (a) F (b) F (c) F (d) T (e) T.

Depressive pseudodementia refers to cognitive impairment
resulting from a depressive illness.   It affects about
10-15% of elderly depressives and resolves with treatment
of the depression.   Pseudodemented patients, in contrast
to demented patients, tend to complain forcibly about
their memory impairment.

References: Post (1982), Rabins et al (1984).

3.25 (a) T (b) T (c) F (d) F (e) T.

Hachinski et al (1975) have developed a scale which
comprises a list of items which indicate that a patient is
more likely to have multi-infarct dementia than Alzheimer
type dementia.   These are: abrupt onset, stepwise
deterioration, fluctuating course, nocturnal confusion,
relative preservation of personality, depression, somatic
complaints, emotional incontinence, history of
hypertension, history of strokes, evidence of associated
atherosclerosis, focal neurological symptoms/signs.

Reference: Hachinski et al (1975).

3.26 (a) T (b) T (c) F (d) F (e) F.

(c) The EEG is abnormal in 90% of patients with a subdural haematoma.

Reference: Lishman (1978).

3.27 (a) F (b) T (c) T (d) T (e) T.

(a) Epileptic automatisms are usually preceded by an aura, the nature of which depends upon the function of the neurones at the site of the focus. Common auras include abdominal sensations, emotional or memory disturbances, vivid recall of the past, hallucinations and gustatory or olfactory phenomena.

(d) While the majority of epileptic automatisms occur with foci in the temporal lobes, they can also occur with foci in the cortex of the frontal and parietal lobes.

Reference: Fenton (1972).

3.28 (a) T (b) T (c) T (d) F (e) T.

(d) The mental disturbances in hepatic encephalopathy are caused by nitrogenous substances which are not metabolised by the damaged liver and are passed into the systemic circulation. High protein intake thus exacerbates the condition.

References: Lunzer (1975), Lishman (1978).

3.29 **(a) T (b) T (c) F (d) T (e) T.**

(a) Serological tests are positive in over 90% of untreated cases of neurosyphilis, but are much more likely to be negative if previous treatment with penicillin has been given. Lumbar puncture is thus indicated when neurosyphilis is suspected but serology is negative.

(b) Dewhurst (1969) found depression to be the most common initial diagnosis in his series of 91 patients with neurosyphilis.

(c) ECT is probably contraindicated in view of reports that it can induce a deterioration with focal neurological signs.

(d) Dementia was the initial diagnosis in 13 of Dewhurst's patients, and is usually present to some degree.

(e) Dysarthria occurs in over 80% of neurosyphilitic patients. Pupillary abnormalities and tremor are other characteristic physical signs.

References: Dewhurst (1969), Lishman (1978).

3.30 **(a) T (b) T (c) T (d) T (e) T.**

Reference: Robertson and Kennedy (1983).

3.31 **(a) F (b) F (c) T (d) T (e) T.**

Trimble (1981) collated several series describing the psychopathology of Huntington's chorea. He found that, in a total sample of 853 patients, 66% had dementia, 17% depression, 9% paranoid states, 8% a schizophreniform illness and 2% were manic.

Reference: Trimble (1981).

3.32 (a) F (b) T (c) F (d) T (e) T.

(a) Kringlen carried out one of the most important twin
studies of schizophrenia.

(b) Lidz and his colleagues suggested that both "schismatic"
marriages, where there were deep irreconcilable
differences between spouses, and "skewed" marriages, in
which one spouse was pathologically dominant over the
other, produced schizophrenic children.

(c) Heston is well known for his studies of children of
schizophrenics who were adopted by non-schizophrenic
parents.

(d) Fromm - Reichman described the "schizophrenogenic mother".

(e) Bateson and his colleagues propounded the "double-bind"
hypothesis as being important in the aetiology of
schizophrenia.

Reference: Wing (1982a).

3.33 (a) T (b) F (c) T (d) F (e) F.

(a) This is thought broadcasting.

(b) This auditory hallucination does not have any of the
special properties of a first rank symptom.

(c) This is a delusional perception.

(d) This resembles a "made action" but the force does not
clearly arise from outside the patient.

(e) This resembles thought insertion, but the thoughts are not
clearly put into the patient's mind.

Reference: Mellor (1970).

3.34 (a) T (b) F (c) T (d) T (e) F.

(a) Torrey et al (1974) found very low rates of schizophrenia in remote tribes who, having had little contact with the Western world, possibly were not exposed to the "virus".

(b) Those in contact with schizophrenics have not been shown to have an increased incidence.

(c) The reduced fertility of schizophrenics suggests that, for it still to be prevalent, it must be a "new" illness, possibly of viral aetiology.

(d) The excess of schizophrenic births in the winter months of the year supports a theory of intrauterine or perinatal infection.

(e) There is no definitive virological or immunological evidence supporting a viral aetiology of schizophrenia.

References: Hare (1979), Crow (1983).

3.35 (a) F (b) F (c) F (d) F (e) F.

(a) Depression occurs in at least a third of chronic schizophrenics.

(b) The contribution of neuroleptics to depression in schizophrenia is small, although patients on very high doses of depot neuroleptics may be more susceptible.

(c) The response of these depressions to tricyclics is disappointingly poor.

Reference: Johnson (1981).

3.36 (a) T (b) F (c) T (d) T (e) F.

(b) While there is probably an association between taking oral contraceptives and minor psychiatric symptoms, there is no convincing evidence indicating an association between their use and frank depressive illness.

Reference: Vessey et al (1985).

3.37 (a) T (b) T (c) T (d) F (e) F.

(e) When auditory hallucinations occur, as they do in about
20% of manic patients, they are almost always consonant
with the elevated mood (e.g. messages from God) and are
thus very rarely threatening. Many writers feel that
psychotic symptoms do not occur in hypomania, by
definition, and when they do the diagnosis is that of
mania.

References: Gibbons (1982), Tyrer and Shopsin (1982).

3.38 (a) F (b) F (c) F (d) F (e) T.

(a) Folie à deux was first described by Lasègue and Falret in
the 1870's, and it involves two people sharing the same
delusional idea, which is usually persecutory or
hypochondriacal.

(c) Although it is sometimes difficult to determine which
partner became deluded first, classically, the delusion
is acquired first by the dominant partner and then adopted
by the submissive one.

(d) Sufferers are usually blood relatives, and most commonly
two sisters are affected. The pair live together and tend
to lead secluded lives.

Reference: Enoch and Trethowan (1979).

3.39 (a) F (b) F (c) F (d) T (e) F.

(a) Puerperal schizophrenia carries a particularly poor prognosis.

(b) Kendell et al (1981) found a sixteen fold increase in the risk of women being admitted with a functional psychosis in the first trimester following childbirth. There is also a substantial increase in the incidence of neurotic depression.

(c), (e) "Maternity blues" peak on days 3 to 5 post-partum, while depressive neurosis is most commonly diagnosed 2 to 3 weeks after delivery. "Maternity blues" are characterised by tearfulness, irritability, insomnia and fatigue, and occur in half to three quarters of women. This usually last only a few days, but severe "blues" can merge into a neurotic depression.

References: Kendell et al (1981), Cox (1983).

3.40 (a) T (b) T (c) T (d) F (e) T.

(a) It is not known why this should be so, although one possibility is the stress associated with migration as rural workers seek employment during this period.

(b) Retrospective studies suggest that over 90% of suicides have suffered from an identifiable mental illness.

(d) Affective illness is the most common psychiatric condition associated with suicide; alcoholism is the second most common condition.

Reference: Kreitman (1983).

3.41 (a) T (b) T (c) F (d) T (c) T.

(c) This disorder, a rare tumour of the medulla of the adrenal gland, causes anxiety, fear, tremor and apprehension. It is, therefore, sometimes misdiagnosed as an anxiety state.

3.42 (a) T (b) F (c) T (d) F (e) F.

(a)   This is an episodic disorder mostly seen among male
      Malays. It is an example of hysterical dissociation in
      which a sudden shock sets off a series of involuntary and
      inappropriate reactions often of an automatic and
      repetitive nature, including echopraxia and echolalia.

(b)   This is a condition associated with narcolepsy, probably
      due to an inborn disorder of metabolism.

(c)   Again, this is a condition found among Malays, and
      involves a sudden outburst of violent rage which may
      result in several homicides and the suicide of the
      perpetrator.

(d)   Capgras' syndrome occurs as a manifestation of a primary
      psychotic disorder, usually schizophrenia. The sufferer
      has a delusional conviction that certain individuals have
      been replaced by their doubles who impersonate them.

(e)   This disorder, associated with visual agnosia, loss of
      fear, and hypersexual behaviour, is caused by temporal
      lobe damage.

Reference: Kräupl Taylor (1983).

3.43 (a) T (b) T (c) T (d) T (e) T.

Reference: Marks (1969), Freeman (1983a).

3.44 (a) T (b) T (c) T (d) T (e) F.

(a)   It may be a symptom of organic brain disease. It may also
      occur as part of the aura in temporal lobe epilepsy.

(c)   Since it often occurs at times of extreme stress, it may
      be a form of defence which allows the individual to cope
      with extreme anxiety.

(e)   It may be a prodromal feature of schizophrenia.

Reference: Snaith (1981).

3.45 (a) T (b) F (c) T (d) T (e) T.

(a) Fugues are usually in response to some immediate threat or stress with which the individual feels unable to cope.

(b) A fugue usually lasts a few hours or days, only occasionally for much longer.

Reference: Kendell (1983b).

3.46 (a) T (b) T (c) F (d) F (e) T.

(c), (d) Serum cholesterol and carotene levels are raised in some patients with anorexia nervosa, for reasons which are not understood.

References: Crisp (1980), Fairburn (1983a).

3.47 (a) T (b) F (c) F (d) F (e) F.

(a) Most studies report normalisation of menstrual function in 50-70% of cases. An early onset of illness is associated with a higher chance of menstruation returning to normal.

(c) The mortality rate is about 5%.

(d), (e) Only about two thirds of patients maintain a normal weight and even fewer have normal eating patterns.

Reference: Steinhausen and Glanville (1983).

3.48 (a) F (b) F (c) T (d) T (e) T.

(a) While exact figures are hard to establish, bulimia nervosa is much commoner than this.

(b) While it is rare in men, it does occur.

(c) Sufferers almost always feel intensely guilty and self-deprecatory after binge-eating.

Reference: Fairburn (1983a).

3.49 (a) F (b) T (c) T (d) T (e) F.

(a) Obsessional individuals keep tight control over their feelings.

(d) In addition to being vulnerable to the development of obsessional neuroses, obsessional personalities are also usually held to be at increased risk of developing agitated depressive illnesses.

Reference: Cooper (1983).

3.50 (a) T (b) T (c) F (d) T (e) T.

(d) Creed (1981) found a significant excess of life events prior to appendicectomy, especially when the appendix removed was histologically normal.

References: Paykel (1978), Ambelas (1979), Creed (1981).

3.51 (a) F (b) T (c) T (d) F (e) F.

(a) Abdominal pain occurs in over 80% of cases.

(b) Stress factors, such as bereavement, and threatening life events, appear to be implicated in the aetiology and maintenance of this disorder.

(d) In European countries the female/male ratio is about 2:1.

(e) It is a disorder of bowel motility. This distinguishes it from other conditions, such as ulcerative colitis, which are inflammatory disorders.

References: Ford et al (1982), Oken (1985).

3.52 (a) T (b) F (c) T (d) F (e) T.

(d) Fetishism in females is very rare, but as yet there is no generally accepted reason why this should be the case.

Reference: Bancroft (1983).

3.53 (a) F (b) F (c) T (d) F (e) F.

(a), (b), (e) Almost all patients with alcoholic hallucinosis
suffer from auditory hallucinations, often of disparaging
voices discussing the patient in the third person. While
the illness can thus be mistaken for schizophrenia, it
persists for less than a week in the great majority of
cases, and there is no significant excess of schizophrenia
in these patients' families.

(c) Alcoholic hallucinations almost always occur when a
patient has substantially reduced his alcohol intake, and
results from the fall in his blood alcohol level. If the
blood alcohol level is restored to its more usual level
with a few drinks, then the hallucinations will be
suppressed.

Reference: Victor (1983).

3.54 (a) F (b) T (c) T (d) F (e) T.

Reference: Edwards and Gross (1976).

3.55 (a) T (b) F (c) T (d) T (e) F.

(b) The babies are irritable, hyperactive, tremulous and sleep
poorly. These symptoms, while resembling those of alcohol
withdrawal, tend to persist.

Reference: Victor (1983).

3.56 (a) F (b) T (c) F (d) F (e) T.

(a) Amphetamines reduce hunger, hence their use in the treatment of obesity.

(b) Amphetamines are central stimulants leading to feelings of euphoria, increased energy, confidence and improved powers of concentration. This arises through their causing central release of noradrenaline and dopamine.

(c), (d), (e) Amphetamine is chemically similar to adrenaline and has weak actions on the sympathetic nervous system leading to tachycardia, hypertension, sweating and palpitations.

Reference: Ghodse (1983).

3.57 (a) T (b) F (c) T (d) T (e) F.

(b) Neurotic and emotional disorders seldom underlie solvent abuse.

(e) There is no firm evidence that solvent abusers have a tendency to progress to harder drugs.

Reference: Sourindrhin (1985).

3.58 (a) F (b) T (c) F (d) T (e) T

Reference: Mezey (1985).

3.59 (a) T (b) F (c) F (d) T (e) F

(a)   If the defence of "diminished responsibility" is accepted
by the jury, a person who would otherwise have been liable
to be convicted of murder is liable instead to be
convicted of manslaughter.

(b), (c)   English law states that a child of under 10 years is
considered to be incapable of forming a guilty intent,
whereas a child of 10-13 years is considered to be capable
of forming a guilty intent if he can distinguish good from
evil.   From the age of 14 years a child in England is
deemed to be fully responsible.   The comparable age in
Scotland is 8 years.

(d), (e)   Certain offences such as indecent assault and
manslaughter do not require proof of guilty intent (mens
rea), whereas others such as murder, rape and arson
require proof of the unlawful act (actus rea) and guilty
intent.

3.60 (a) F (b) T (c) T (d) T (e) F.

(a), (e)   Wernicke (1848-1905) was a major contributor to
German neuropsychiatry and provided the first systematic
description of sensory aphasia.   Beard (1839-1883) made
popular the term "neuraesthenia".

(b)   Cullen (1710- 1790) coined the term "neurosis" to describe
a variety of disorders of the nervous system in which
there was no fever.

(c)   Morel (1809-1873) introduced the concept of "démence
précoce" which was later incorporated into Kraepelin's
classification of dementia praecox.

(d)   Sydenham (1624-1689) provided detailed descriptions of
hysteria and its psychological and physiological aspects,
distinguishing it from other disorders.

Reference: Bynum (1983).

PAPER 4 – ANSWERS

4.1 (a) F (b) T (c) T (d) F (e) T.

(a) Traumatic mutism is preceded by a psychological or
     physical trauma. Elective mutism is usually restricted to
     a particular setting or to a particular group of
     intimates.

(d) Compared to other nonpsychotic, nonorganic psychiatric
     disorders of childhood, elective mutism is rather
     resistant to treatment.

Reference: Kolvin (1983).

4.2 (a) F (b) T (c) T (d) F (e) F.

(a) They are at least twice as common in boys.

(c) It is uncommon for tics to appear for the first time in
     adulthood.

(d) They are unrelated to intelligence.

(e) They usually last only a few weeks or months. Only about
     10% of cases continue into adulthood.

Reference: Corbett (1983).

4.3 (a) F (b) T (c) T (d) T (e) T.

(a) Children of immigrant families (especially West Indians) have a higher rate of conduct disorder, possibly due to such factors as larger family size, their attendance at schools with a high rate of pupil turnover, and their raised rates of educational retardation.

(b) The prevalence among children with chronic or recurrent physical illness is twice as high as that among healthy children.

Reference: Wolff (1983).

4.4 (a) T (b) F (c) F (d) F (e) F.

(a) Although few of the studies are free of methodological difficulties, it is virtually certain that there is a significant genetic component to the aetiology of specific reading retardation.

Reference: Yule and Rutter (1985).

4.5 (a) T (b) T (c) T (d) F (e) T.

(d) Tricyclics provide complete relief in about one third of bed wetters, but wetting often returns when the drug is stopped.

(e) Drinking before bedtime can help the child to "overlearn" the relationship between a full bladder, micturition and the alarm.

References: Berg (1981), Wolff (1983b).

4.6 (a) F (b) T (c) T (d) F (e) F.

(a) Traditionally, the middle years of childhood have been described as a "latent" period, with little interest in sexual matters. This is incorrect. Although prepubertal children play almost exclusively with their own sex, heterosexual interests are popular and extensive.

(d) Animal phobias are common among preschool children, whereas social phobia and agoraphobia are rare before puberty and are more likely than animal phobias to emerge during adolescence.

(e) Delinquency rises to a peak in the mid teens, and diminishes sharply in early adult life.

Reference: Graham and Rutter (1985).

4.7 (a) F (b) T (c) T (d) F (e) T.

(a) About 30% of autistic children will develop epilepsy.

(b), (c) Kanner originally believed that autistic children were of normal or even superior intelligence, but at least 50% are seriously retarded with IQ's below 50. Moreover, there is no evidence to suggest that the children's intellectual function is artificially depressed by their psychotic state.

(d) Despite earlier unsubstantiated claims, there are no grounds for believing that autism is a product of parental rejection, lack of maternal warmth or other deficiencies of parenting.

(e) Estimates of prevalence vary, but autism probably occurs in about 4.5 per 10,000 children between the ages of 8-10 years, with a 3:1 ratio of boys to girls.

Reference: Reid (1982).

4.8 (a) F (b) T (c) F (d) T (e) F.

(a)   The figure is higher at about 6/1000.

Reference: Murray and McGuffin (1983).

4.9 (a) T (b) F (c) T (d) T (c) F.

(a), (b), (c), (d)   This infantile form of cerebro-macular
    degeneration appears to be an autosomal recessive disorder
    which is particularly common in Jews. It is associated
    with increased lipid storage throughout the central
    nervous system, including in the retinal ganglion cells
    resulting in progressive blindness. Spasticity, apathy,
    weakness and mental retardation are typical features.
    Death is common before 4 years.

(e)   Tuberous sclerosis (epiloia) causes a facial "butterfly
    rash".

Reference: Zealley (1983).

4.10 (a) T (b) T (c) T (d) F (e) F.

(a), (b) It has long been accepted that Down's patients show a
high vulnerability to Alzheimer's disease. This may be
associated with their vulnerability also to affective
illness in that the latter may be a prodromal sign of the
impending dementing process.

(c) Although autistic children initially have a higher risk of
epilepsy than do Down's patients, as the latter age their
risk of developing epilepsy increases. This fact may be
related to the progressive neurological changes associated
with Alzheimer's disease.

(d) In childhood, Down's patients are frequently reported as
cheerful and largely cooperative at home but this is not
so true of those who reach late adolescence and adult
life : behavioural problems become much more common and
institutional care may become necessary.

(e) Echolalia is a normal feature of language development, and
therefore its presence may merely indicate incomplete
language development.

Reference: Reid (1982).

4.11 (a) F (b) T (c) T (d) T (e) T.

The Therapeutic Community movement was initiated by
Maxwell Jones as a reaction against the undesirable
effects of large institutions. Patients in such
communities are encouraged to take responsibility for
their own actions and to face up to realities. The milieu
is one of democracy and freedom.

References: Jones (1976), Clark (1977).

4.12 (a) T (b) T (c) T (d) F (e) F.

(a) Reinforcing stimuli may be presented either according to certain time intervals or response frequencies.

(c) In "shaping", the organism is rewarded when it behaves in a way progressively similar to the desired final response.

(d) I P Pavlov (1849-1936), a Russian physiologist, pioneered research into classical conditioning.

(e) In operant conditioning, reinforcement is presented <u>only</u> if the desired behavior is "emitted" by the subject.

4.13 (a) T (b) T (c) F (d) T (e) F.

Bion distinguished between two aspects of a group - the "work group" and the "basic assumption group". The former refers to the ostensible purpose of the group; the latter refers to tacit assumptions within the group which prevent it fulfilling that purpose. He recognized 3 "basic assumption groups" : the "pairing group" (when members become preoccupied with pairings), the "fight/flight group" (when members are preparing to fight or flee), and the "dependency group" (when strivings for dependency may predominate).

(c) Encounter groups developed from the National Training Laboratories, an organization established in 1947 by social psychologists. These groups encourage the uninhibited expression of emotions, often involving physical contact.

(d) T-groups (training groups) emphasize training in self-awareness and group dynamics.

References: Bion (1961), Rioch (1970).

4.14 (a) F (b) T (c) F (d) F (e) T.

(a)   The Premack Principle states that an activity or behaviour
may be reinforced by engaging in other behaviour of
greater baseline frequency.

(b)   Biofeedback usually involves the use of electrical
monitoring devices which detect and amplify internal
physiological processes, many of which are generally
regarded as being otherwise beyond conscious control.   In
other instances the function may be normally under
consious control but this has failed for some reason, as
is the case with faecal incontinence.   Biofeedback makes
available to the patient information about the state of
the processes, thereby providing an opportunity for
gaining or regaining some degree of control over them.

(d)   Although no single individual can be accredited with
"devising" biofeedback, this procedure owes much to the
pioneering efforts of Di Cara and Miller in the USA in the
1950's and 1960's.   They showed that the autonomic nervous
system could be brought under at least some degree of
conscious control.

(e)   In analogue feedback the information varies continuously
and changes directly with alterations in the system being
monitored.   Binary feedback provides only "on/off"
feedback, confirming that the feature being monitored is
either above or below a predetermined criterion.

References: Johnston (1978), Kogeorgos and Scott (1981).

4.15   (a) T (b) T (c) T (d) T (e) T.

Abreaction can occur in response to a variety of factors
including sudden noises, psychotherapy, psychodrama, and
hypnosis.   The process and outcome of abreaction are
similar irrespective of the way in which it has been
induced.

Reference: Marks (1982).

4.16 (a) F (b) F (c) T (d) T (e) T.

(a)   Beck is associated with Cognitive Behavioural therapy.

(b)   Ellis is associated with Rational-Emotive therapy; Bandura
      is associated with modelling.

4.17 (a) T (b) T (c) T (d) F (e) T.

(d)   If anything, more unilateral treatments are required to
      produce the same response.

Reference: Freeman (1983c).

4.18 (a) T (b) T (c) F (d) T (e) T.

      The symptoms of benzodiazepine withdrawal can be seen in
      terms of "rebound phenomena", representing the reverse
      effects from those produced by the drug.

Reference: Tyrer (1982a).

4.19 (a) F (b) T (c) T (d) T (e) T.

Reference: Loudon (1983).

4.20 (a) F (b) T (c) F (d) T (e) F.

(a)   L-tryptophan has a short plasma half-life and should thus
      be taken three or four times per day.

(c)   It is safe and often efficacious in combination with
      tricyclics.

(d)   L-tryptophan is metabolised to 5-HT of which 5HIAA is a
      degradation product.

(e)   It has no effect on noradrenergic neurones.

References: Tyrer (1982b), Loudon (1983).

4.21 (a) F (b) T (c) T (d) F (e) T.

(a) Although medical use of lithium dates back to the mid-19th century, credit for its first psychiatric usage is usually given to Cade, who used it on manic patients in Australia in the late 1940's.

(b) Lithium inhibits the formation of cyclic AMP through its effect on the enzyme adenylate cyclase, and this is responsible for its effects on the thyroid gland and kidney function.

(d) Administration of lithium in the first trimester of pregnancy is almost certainly associated with increased rates of foetal abnormalities, especially malformations of the cardiovascular system. If it is decided to continue lithium during pregnancy, then serum lithium levels should be kept as low as possible. Lithium crosses the placenta freely and neonatal lithium toxicity may occur without maternal blood levels having reached the toxic range.

(e) Mothers on lithium should usually be discouraged from breast feeding, due to the risk of toxicity in the baby.

References: Weinstein (1980), Tyrer and Shaw (1982).

4.22 (a) T (b) F (c) T (d) T (e) F.

(b) Retinitis pigmentosa occurs with thioridazine, especially when it is given in doses above 800mg/day.

Reference: Mackay (1982).

4.23　(a) F (b) F (c) T (d) F (e) F.

(a)　It is a phenothiazine.

(b)　It is among the most sedative of the neuroleptics.

(c), (d)　On account of its propensity to block cholinergic receptors, thioridazine produces Parkinsonism more rarely than other neuroleptics.

(e)　Prolactin levels are raised due to blockade of dopamine receptors in the anterior pituitary.

Reference:　Mackay (1982).

4.24　(a) F (b) F (c) F (d) T (e) F.

(a), (b)　Neurotic illnesses, although not widely studied in the elderly, are almost certainly less common than in younger patients and tend to decline further in prevalence with increasing old age.

(c)　Females are affected about 5 times more often than men.

(e)　Bergmann (1971), in a community survey, found that while many elderly neurotics had long-standing illnesses and/or predisposing personality traits, about half of such patients became neurotically ill after the age of 60.

References:　Bergmann (1971), Kay (1976), Post (1982).

4.25   (a) T (b) F (c) F (d) F (e) F.

(a)   There is an approximately four-fold increase in the risk of senile dementia in first degree relatives.

(b), (c)   The life expectancy of demented elderly patients is considerably reduced, although their survival time after entering hospital care is significantly longer than it was 30 years ago.

(d)   About 80% of the demented elderly are cared for in the community.

(e)   Demented elderly people who live alone are at much the greatest risk of requiring institutional care.

References: Bergmann (1975), Bergmann et al (1978), Christie and Train (1984).

4.26   (a) F (b) F (c) T (d) F (e) T.

(a), (b), (d)   These symptoms are more common as early features of Alzheimer's disease since it tends to cause greatest damage to the parietal lobes.

(c), (e)   These features arise due to the propensity of Pick's disease to have greatest effect on the frontal lobes.

Reference: Lishman (1978).

4.27 (a) F (b) T (c) T (d) F (e) T.

(a) The overall incidence is very similar in men and women.

(b) There is a significant genetic contribution to the aetiology of epilepsy, especially that of the "idiopathic" type.

(c) This probably occurs due to the condition itself and to the availability of barbiturates.

(d) Even in late onset epilepsy, tumour is a relatively rare cause.

Reference: Lishman (1978).

4.28 (a) F (b) F (c) T (d) T (e) T.

(a) Regular consumption of large amounts of alcohol over more then ten years is usually held to be required to produce alcoholic dementia, while bout drinking is less harmful.

(e) Radiological abnormalities – cortical atrophy and ventricular enlargement – can be demonstrated in about two thirds of alcoholic in-patients.

Reference: Cutting (1982).

4.29 (a) T (b) T (c) T (d) F (e) F.

(a) About 6 women are affected for every man.

(c) Very rarely, "apathetic hyperthyroidism" occurs, when the patient suffers from apathy and inertia.

(e) The most usual differential diagnosis of hyperthyroidism is from anxiety neurosis. In both disorders, weight loss is common, but while appetite tends to be reduced in anxiety states, it is usually increased in hyperthyroidism.

Reference: Lishman (1978).

4.30 (a) T (b) F (c) T (d) F (e) T.

Surridge (1969) studied 108 patients with multiple
sclerosis. About a quarter were euphoric, about a quarter
were depressed and about two thirds showed intellectual
impairment. There was a high correlation between euphoria
and intellectual impairment.

References: Surridge (1969), Lishman (1978).

4.31 (a) T (b) F (c) T (d) F (e) F.

(b) An indistinguishable syndrome occurs without neuroleptics,
almost always in the elderly.

(d), (e) Tardive dyskinesia probably reflects relative
dopaminergic overactivity in the nigrostriatal tract
(usually secondary to prolonged dopaminergic blockade),
coupled with relative cholinergic underactivity.
Anticholinergic medication is thus likely to worsen the
condition. Indeed, since there is no effective treatment
for tardive dyskinesia, the emphasis rests on prevention.
This comprises using the minimum effective dose of a
neuroleptic for the briefest praticable period and
remaining vigilant for the condition, particularly in
older patients.

Reference: Mackay (1982).

4.32 (a) F (b) T (c) T (d) T (e) F.

Bleuler considered the primary symptoms of schizophrenia
to comprise the "four A's" of ambivalence, autism,
affective blunting and associative loosening.

(a) Apophany is synonomous with a primary delusional
experience.

4.33 (a) F (b) T (c) T (d) F (e) F.

(a) These conditions do coexist and in Parkinson's disease there is a relative <u>depletion</u> of dopamine activity.

(b) Amphetamines induce the release of dopamine and inhibit its reuptake, and can produce a syndrome indistinguishable from schizophrenia.

(c) Haloperidol, like other neuroleptics, blocks dopamine receptors.

(d) HVA is a metabolite of dopamine and its CSF level tends to be normal or low in schizophrenia.

(e) Dopamine inhibits prolactin release, but prolactin levels in schizophrenics have not been shown to be abnormal.

Reference: Iversen (1978).

4.34 (a) F (b) T (c) T (d) T (e) F.

(a), (e) Prolixity (a more ordered form of flight of ideas) and clang associations (rhyming associations between words) are characteristic of hypomania.

Reference: Hamilton (1985).

4.35 (a) F (b) T (c) F (d) T (e) F.

References: Vaillant (1964), Stephens et al (1966).

4.36 (a) T (b) T (c) T (d) F (e) F.

(a)   The prognosis is intermediate between that of affective
      psychosis and schizophrenia.

(b), (c) While there is an increased incidence of both
      disorders in relatives, the incidence of affective
      psychosis has usually been found to be higher than that of
      schizophrenia.

(e)   The term "schizo-affective" was coined by Kasanin. Magnan
      introduced the term "bouffée délirante"

Reference: Kendell (1983c).

4.37 (a) T (b) T (c) T (d) T (e) T.

Delusions of poverty, sinfulness, disease, guilt,
worthlessness and nihilistic delusions are "classical"
depressive delusions. While being less specific to
depression, delusions of persecution and reference are
just as common.

4.38 (a) T (b) T (c) F (d) F (e) F.

(c)   Women are affected about twice as often as men which
      favours the X-linked theory of inheritance.

(d)   Father to son transmission does occur, providing strong
      evidence against the theory.

(e)   A few studies have demonstrated linkage between manic
      depressive illness and the colour blindness region of the
      X-chromosome. It seems probable that X-linked inheritance
      does occur in a small minority of manic depressive
      families.

References: Murray and McGuffin (1983), Del Zompo (1984).

4.39 (a) F (b) T (c) F (d) F (e) F.

(a) The majority of women benefit psychologically from
hysterectomy, with improvement of mood and social and
psychosexual functioning.

(b) Gath et al (1982a,b) found that 29% of 148 women were
"cases" on the PSE 18 months after hysterectomy.

(e) Gath et al found that, if there is a relationship between
age and psychological outcome, then younger women tend to
do rather better.

References: Coppen et al (1981), Gath et al (1982a,b).

4.40 (a) F (b) T (c) T (d) F (e) T.

(a) Parasuicide rather than suicide is predominant among young
people between 15 and 25 years.

(b) In terms of marital status, the highest rates of suicide
are for the divorced, followed by the single and widowed.

(d) The suicide rate drops during war but returns to the
pre-war level on the cessation of hostilities.

Reference: Kreitman (1983).

4.41 (a) F (b) T (c) F (d) T (e) F.

(a), (c) Psychotic rather than neurotic depression is
associated with nihilistic delusions and a high risk of
suicide.

Reference: Goldberg (1983).

4.42 (a) T (b) T (c) T (d) F (e) F.

(a) Problems of definition and selection have led to a variety of epidemiological findings but the consensus is that, among the neuroses, obsessional ones are uncommon.

(c) Seventy-five per cent of such neuroses occur before the age of 30 years. Few cases begin after 50 years of age.

(e) The identification of precipitating factors is difficult, but current evidence suggests that only in about 50 per cent of cases are there precipitating events, such as illness, bereavement or other life changes.

Reference: Cooper (1983).

4.43 (a) T (b) T (c) T (d) F (e) F.

Reference: Gelder (1983).

4.44 (a) T (b) T (c) T (d) F (e) F.

(d) In dissociative states the EEG is one of full consciousness; sleep talking can occur during any stage of sleep.

(e) In this syndrome (also known as "erotomania" and "psychose passionelle") a woman suffers from a delusion that a man, usually older than she is and of higher social status, is in love with her.

Reference: Ellis (1985).

4.45 (a) F (b) T (c) T (d) F (e) F.

(b) The incidence of parasuicide among pathological gamblers is over 8 times that of the general population.

(d) Although the initial response is quite good, the relapse rate is disappointing.

Reference: Moran (1983).

4.46 (a) T (b) F (c) T (d) F (e) F.

(a), (b), (c) Cortisol levels tend to be raised and as many as
70% of anorexics show a pattern of non-suppression on the
DST. ADH levels are usually low. These parameters tend
to normalise with weight gain.

(d), (e) CSF noradrenaline, homovanilic acid (a metabolite of
dopamine) and 5-HIAA (a metabolite of 5-HT) are all
reduced in underweight anorexics. While HVA and 5-HIAA
levels normalise with weight gain, CSF noradrenaline seems
to remain low in recovered anorexics.

References: Fichter et al (1982), Gold et al (1983), Kaye et
al (1984).

4.47 (a) T (b) T (c) F (d) T (e) F.

(c) The theory that anorexia nervosa represents an atypical
affective disorder was probably first advanced by
Cantwell.

(d) Bruch feels that the anorexic's "paralysing sense of
ineffectiveness" is one of the causes of the desperate
control she seeks'to establish over her eating and her
weight.

(e) This is an extreme behavioural view of aetiology: Crisp
adopts an eclectic view of the disorder which leans
towards psychodynamic theories of aetiology.

Reference: Hsu (1983).

4.48 **(a) T (b) T (c) T (d) T (e) T.**

(a) Amenorrhoea or oligomenorrhoea is quite common in bulimia nervosa, while not being invariable as they are in anorexia nervosa.

(b) This is probably a result of the hypokalaemia arising from vomiting and purgative abuse.

(c), (d) These arise from repeated regurgitation of acidic gastric contents.

Reference: Fairburn (1983b).

4.49 **(a) F (b) T (c) F (d) T (e) F.**

(a) As a group, psychopaths tend to have at least average IQ.

(c) The high rates of neurotic symptoms in patients diagnosed as psychopathic have led some authors to consider such patients as "acting-out neurotics", indicating that these individuals tolerate anxiety poorly and respond to it by behaving aggressively.

(d) A high proportion of psychopaths, primarily those who are aggressive and impulsive, have "immature" EEGs similar to those of children.

(e) In learning tasks, psychopaths tend to acquire conditioned responses more slowly than normal people. It is hypothesised that this slow learning underlies their maladaptive behaviour, in that it explains their apparently impaired ability to learn the usual "social rules". The term "sociopathic" is based on this hypothesis, as is the treatment of psychopaths in therapeutic communities where they can attempt to "learn" socially acceptable conduct.

References: Whitely (1970), Freeman (1983).

4.50 (a) T (b) F (c) T (d) F (e) F.

(c) Although the exact association between insomnia and apnoea is not clear, obese males under 40 years are most affected.

(d) The disturbed sleep found in old age is associated with diminished amounts of slow-wave sleep (stages 3 and 4).

(e) Nicotine is a powerful stimulant. Smoking is also associated with respiratory problems and thus coughing and impaired respiration may keep smokers awake.

Reference: Oswald (1983).

4.51 (a) T (b) T (c) F (d) T (e) T.

Reference: Bond (1979).

4.52 (a) T (b) T (c) F (d) F (e) F.

(c), (d) The sexes are affected equally, although schizophrenia in males tends to appear earlier than in females.

(e) It is more common in males.

4.53 (a) F (b) T (c) F (d) F (e) T

(a) Its real incidence has not been established but among patient samples male transsexuals are at least twice as common as females.

(b) Transvestites obtain sexual pleasure from "cross-dressing".

Reference: Christie-Brown (1983).

4.54 (a) T (b) F (c) T (d) T (e) T.

(b)   The affect is typically labile, and is often elated, perplexed or fearful.

(c), (d), (e)   The autonomic nervous system is characteristically overactive in delirium tremens, this feature serving to distinguish it from nonalcoholic forms of delirium.

Reference: Victor (1983).

4.55 (a) F (b) T (c) F (d) F (e) T.

(a)   Disulfiram inhibits the enzyme acetaldehyde dehydrogenase, leading to toxic levels of acetaldehyde when alcohol is ingested, and hence to the unpleasant effects of the "disulfiram – ethanol reaction".

(c)   The "disulfiram–ethanol reaction" can occur up to 80 hours after the last dose of disulfiram.

(d)   Hypotension is induced.

Reference: Thorley (1982).

4.56 (a) F (b) T (c) T (d) T (e) T.

(a), (b)   Tolerance does develop to amphetamine–induced euphoria, to its cardiovascular effects and to its appetite suppressant effects.   Only very limited tolerance develops to its awakening effects, however, thus making it an effective treatment for narcolepsy.

Reference: Ghodse (1983).

4.57 (a) T (b) F (c) T (d) F (e) T.

(a) The mortality rate is over 20 times that of the rate
expected for a non-dependent population of similar
characteristics. The cause of death is usually drug
overdose of opiates and/or of other injected drugs,
particularly barbiturates.

(c) This arises as a result of serum hepatitis, which is
relatively common in those who abuse intravenous drugs.

(e) Acute pulmonary oedema and angiothrombotic pulmonary
hypertension can be caused by intravenous injection of the
inert material added to the capsules or tablets.

Reference: Ghodse (1983).

4.58 (a) F (b) T (c) F (d) F (e) T.

(a) Menopausal symptoms are no more common among female
shop-lifters than among other women of similar age.
Although middle-aged women do have a high rate compared to
women in other age groups, this may largely reflect the
high proportion of women of this age group among shoppers.

(b) In adults the female to male ratio is approximately 5:2
but in juveniles the sexes are equally represented among
shoplifters.

(d) There is no proven association between pregnancy and
shoplifting.

Reference: Fisher (1984).

4.59 (a) T (b) T (c) T (d) T (e) T.

A trial of fitness to plead is held before a special jury.
If the individual is declared unfit to plead then he is
admitted to a Special Hospital until fit to do so, as
decided by the Home Secretary.

4.60 **(a) T (b) T (c) T (d) F (e) T.**

(a)   Freud studied under Bernheim who viewed the capacity to be hypnotized as quite normal (in contrast to Charcot).

(c)   The word "hypnosis" was coined by Braid, a 19th Century physician.

(d)   Cerletti was a pioneer of electro-convulsive therapy.

(e)   Elliotson, a president of the Royal Medical and Chirurgical Society of London, championed in the 19th century the use of hypnosis as a means of achieving analgesia and anaesthesia.

Reference: Gibson   (1977).

PAPER 5 - ANSWERS

5.1 (a) T (b) F (c) F (d) F (e) T.

(b) Nocturnal enuresis can occur at any stage of the sleep
cycle.

(d) Urinary tract infection is present in about 5% of
enuretics, and is much more common in female than in male
enuretics.

(e) Rutter's large study on the Isle of Wight found rates for
9-10 year olds of 2.9% in boys and 2.2% in girls. This
had fallen to 1.1% and 0.5% respectively by the age of 14.

Reference: Shaffer (1985).

5.2 (a) T (b) T (c) F (d) T (e) T.

(c) A follow-up study over two and a quarter years of children
with head injuries showed that there was a marked increase
in psychiatric disorder only following severe head injury
(ie that resulting in post-traumatic amnesia of at least 7
days). Mild head injury (ie that resulting in post-
traumatic amnesia of less than 7 days) showed no such
increase.

(d) The most rapid period of recovery occurred in the first
few months after injury, but significant recovery
continued for a year, with some improvement continuing
into the second year - especially among those with severe
head injuries.

References: Chadwick et al (1981), Brown et al (1981).

5.3 (a) T (b) F (c) T (d) F (e) F.

(a), (c) The majority of insect and animal phobias start
before the age of 5 years.

(b) The peaks of onset for agoraphobia are in late adolescence
and around the age of 30 years.

(d) Social phobias come on at or after puberty.

(e) Specific situational phobias can begin at any time; height
phobias are not particularly common in children of any
age.

Reference: Hersov (1985a).

5.4 (a) F (b) T (c) F (d) T (e) T.

(b), (c) Adolescent boys are slower than girls to develop
heterosexual interests and activities, but they are more
likely than girls to have a variety of sexual partners.

Reference: Graham and Rutter (1985).

5.5 (a) T (b) T (c) T (d) T (e) F.

(a) Boys are affected three times more often than girls.

(b) The mean age of diagnosis is about 7 years, with a range
of 2 to 15 years. Tics, which are almost always the first
feature, are usually present for a year or two before the
diagnosis is made.

(e) IQ is normally distributed.

Reference: Corbett and Turpin (1985).

5.6 (a) F (b) T (c) F (d) T (e) F.

(a) It has proved difficult to establish precise estimates of incidence but a reasonable estimate is that school refusal accounts for about 5% of all children referred for psychiatric problems. There is a higher rate in secondary schools than in infant or primary schools.

(c) Although an acute onset is more common among younger children, in older children and adolescents the development is more likely to be gradual.

(e) Precipitating factors, such as loss of friends or illness, can be identified quite frequently.

Reference: Hersov (1985b).

5.7 (a) T (b) F (c) T (d) T (e) T.

(a) The risk for such mothers is about 1/50.

(b) A small number of children have a translocation of additional chromosome 21 material.

Reference: Murray and McGuffin (1983).

5.8 (a) T (b) T (c) T (d) F (e) T.

(a) Tay-Sach's disease is a deficiency in a specific hexosaminidase.

(b) Galactosaemia is a disorder of carbohydrate metabolism.

(c) Hartnup's disease involves the defective metabolism of tryptophan.

(d) Klinefelter's syndrome is a chromosomal anomaly (XXY or XXXY).

(e) Phenylketonuria is due to a deficiency or impairment of the enzyme phenylalanine hydroxylase.

5.9 (a) T (b) F (c) T (d) F (e) F.

(b) Phenylketonuria is caused by a deficiency of this enzyme.

(d) Phenylalanine is an essential aminoacid and a dietary minimum is thus required.

(e) It is a blood test.

Reference: Zealley (1983).

5.10 (a) F (b) F (c) F (d) T (e) F.

Reference: Russell (1985).

5.11 (a) F (b) T (c) F (d) F (e) T.

(a) In flooding, the patient is exposed to the feared object without relaxation training and avoidance is prevented.

(c) In response prevention, sometimes used for obsessive – compulsive neurosis, the patient is prevented from displaying or carrying out the maladaptive behaviour.

(d) Modelling refers to the acquisition of new behaviour by imitation.

Reference: Rimm and Masters (1979).

5.12 (a) T (b) T (c) F (d) T (e) T.

(c) This term was used by Anna Freud to refer to those occasions when the patient's transference feelings spilled over into situations outside of therapy. Thus, for instance, feelings about the therapist would be enacted towards other people in the patient's life.

Reference: Sandler et al (1970).

5.13 (a) T (b) T (c) T (d) F (e) T.

(d) Carl Rogers developed client—centred therapy (an example of the humanist — existential school of psychotherapy).

Reference: Gurman and Kniskern (1981).

5.14 (a) F (b) T (c) F (d) T (e) F.

(a) The conditioned stimulus must be presented either at the same time as or slightly before the unconditioned stimulus. In Pavlov's original studies the bell had to be presented at the same time as or slightly before the food to ensure the dogs salivated later to the bell on its own.

(c) E L Thorndike (1874 — 1949) introduced the Law of Effect which states that if a behaviour is followed by a reward it will become more probable under similar conditions.

(e) "Successive approximations" is a term associated with operant or instrumental conditioning whereby the organism is rewarded whenever it behaves in a way which is increasingly similar to the desired response.

5.15 (a) F (b) F (c) T (d) F (e) F.

The term was coined by Eric Berne, the founder of Transactional Analysis. He described three such states: the Parent, the Adult and the Child, each referring to a particular system of feelings and thoughts, and to a related set of behaviour patterns. The term "strokes" was introduced by him to describe the basic motivating factors of human behaviour. A "complementary transaction" refers to a particular stimulus from the Ego—state of one person and the corresponding response from the same Ego—state of another individual.

Reference: Berne (1964).

5.16 **(a) F (b) T (c) T (d) F (e) F.**

(a)   The patient is encouraged to evaluate accurately his attributes in order to to alter his negative view of himself.

(d)   "Contingency contracting" is a technique used in marital therapy.

(e)   Lewin's Field Theory was concerned with an individual's dynamics in relation to the social forces around him.

Reference: Beck (1976).

5.17 **(a) T (b) F (c) T (d) T (e) T.**

(b)   One would require to persevere with full doses of antidepressants for at least 21 days before giving ECT on the basis that the patient has "failed to respond".

(d), (e)   The presence of delusions was found in the Northwich Park trial to be the only predictor of a good response to ECT in depressed patients.

References: Freeman (1983c), Clinical Research Centre (1984).

5.18 **(a) T (b) F (c) F (d) F (e) T.**

Chlordiazepoxide and other benzodiazepines raise the fit threshold. In the case of a patient who does not have a fit following the administration of ECT it is worthwhile ventilating him with pure oxygen beforehand and/or premedicating with a phenothiazine, as well as stopping concurrent benzodiazepines.

Reference: Freeman (1983c).

5.19 **(a) T (b) T (c) T (d) F (e) F.**

Reference: Tyrer (1982b).

5.20 (a) F (b) T (c) T (d) T (e) F.

(a) If anything, clomipramine causes more severe unwanted
    effects.

(b) Clomipramine is one of the most specific inhibitors of
     5-HT reuptake.

(c) While clomipramine is often used in obsessional states, it
     is probable that its therapeutic efficacy in such
     conditions depends upon its effect on coexisting
     depression.

References: Marks et al (1980), Mindham (1982).

5.21 (a) T (b) T (c) F (d) T (e) F.

(a), (e) The effects of withdrawal from diazepam are less
          severe because the active metabolites of the drug remain
          in the bloodstream for over four days, while oxazepam is
          eliminated much more rapidly. Withdrawal symptoms can be
          ameliorated by substituting benzodiazepines with longer
          half-lives (such as diazepam) for those with shorter
          half-lives(such as oxazepam) prior to discontinuing the
          drug.

(b) Withdrawal effects seldom arise in patients who have had
     benzodiazepines for less than three months.

(c) Symptoms quite commonly persist for over 3 weeks, and for
     up to 6 weeks.

Reference: Tyrer (1982a).

5.22   (a) F (b) T (c) F (d) F (e) T.

(a)   It is a butyrophenone.

(d)   Its plasma half-life is longer at 12 to 38 hours.

(e)   Milligram for milligram, haloperidol is many times more potent than chlorpromazine.

Reference: Mackay (1982).

5.23   (a) F (b) T (c) F (d) F (e) T.

(c)   Intramuscular procyclidine is nearly always required, especially as the dystonia is very distressing to the patient and requires rapid relief.

(d)   Younger patients are more commonly affected.

Reference: Mackay (1982).

5.24   (a) F (b) F (c) T (d) F (e) T.

(a)   Women are affected about 5 times more commonly than men.

(b)   While the exact frequency of first-rank symptoms in late paraphrenia is a matter of current debate, they occur in at least 30% of patients.

(c)   About 40% are deaf.

References: Grahame (1982, 1984), Post (1982).

5.25 (a) T (b) T (c) F (d) F (e) T.

(c) The EEG is always abnormal, with slow waves and reduced alpha rhythm.

(d), (e) These enzymes, involved in the synthesis and metabolism of acetyl choline, are both reduced in Alzheimer's disease, reflecting the loss of cholinergic neurones which occurs.

References: Folstein and McHugh (1983), Robertson and Kennedy (1983).

5.26 (a) F (b) T (c) F (d) T (e) T.

(a) Many patients improve over the course of years rather than months and a firm prognosis should probably not be offered, except for the most serious injuries, until about three years have elapsed from the time of injury.

(c) Epilepsy arises after about 5% of closed head injuries and after about 30% of penetrating head injuries.

Reference: Lishman (1973).

5.27 (a) T (b) F (c) T (d) T (e) T.

Reference: Lishman (1978).

5.28 (a) T (b) T (c) F (d) T (e) T.

(a), (c), (e) External rectus paralysis is the other common "eye sign" in Wernicke's encephalopathy.

Reference: Robertson and Kennedy (1983).

5.29 (a) T (b) F (c) F (d) T (e) F

(a)   As is the case after other causes of cerebral anoxia, although normal health can apparently be regained for days or even weeks, this can be followed by an acute relapse with delirium and extrapyramidal disturbances.

(b)   Since the detoxification of domestic gas, carbon monoxide poisoning has become a less common method of suicide.

(d)   Nearly half of patients surviving carbon monoxide poisoning will incur cognitive deficits, although severe neuropsychiatric damage occurs in only about 10% of cases. The likelihood of such sequelae correlates with the level of consciousness on admission to hospital.

(e)   Parkinsonism is a rare complication.

Reference: Lishman (1978).

5.30 (a) F (b) T (c) F (d) T (e) T.

It seems almost certain that only a minority of patients with vitamin B12 deficiency have organic mental impairment. Indeed, Elwood et al (1971) in a community survey of over 500 old people found no association between low vitamin B12 (or low folate levels) and impairment on cognitive testing. While associated mild dysmnesic syndromes tend to respond to hydroxycobalamin, established dementias do not.

References: Shulman (1967), Elwood et al (1971), Robertson and Kennedy (1983).

5.31 (a) T (b) F (c) T (d) F (e) F.

(b) Women are clinically affected more often than men in a
ratio of about 3:2.

(c) People not infrequently carry the gene for AIP while
remaining phenotypically normal.

(d) Onset is usually between puberty and middle age.

(e) Transmission is by a Mendelian dominant gene.

Reference: Robertson and Kennedy (1983).

5.32 (a) T (b) T (c) F (d) F (e) T.

Reference: Mellor (1970).

5.33 (a) T (b) T (c) F (d) F (e) T.

(d) Relatives more often direct criticism at what they
perceive to be the patient's personality.

References: Brown et al (1972), Vaughn and Leff (1976).

5.34 (a) T (b) F (c) T (d) F (e) F.

(b) The lifetime risk is about 10%.

(d) The genetically inherited propensity to develop
schizophrenia is almost certainly polygenically
determined.

(e) Age of separation of a child from a schizophrenic parent
has not been shown to have any effect on that child's
chances of developing schizophrenia.

Reference: Shields (1978).

5.35 **(a) T (b) F (c) F (d) F (e) T.**

5.36 **(a) F (b) F (c) F (d) T (e) T.**

(a) In Capgras' syndrome the patient is delusionally convinced that someone, usually a close relative, has been replaced by a double.

(b) "Mirror gazing" usually occurs in anorexia nervosa and in Alzheimer's disease.

(c), (d) Capgras' syndrome does occur in organic states, such as after head injury, but it much more commonly occurs in the functional psychoses.

Reference: Enoch and Trethowan (1979).

5.37 **(a) T (b) F (c) F (d) T (e) T.**

(b) The premorbid personalities of bipolar patients tend to be more extraverted as well as less tense and anxious than those of unipolar patients.

(c) While Perris (1966) found that episodes of illness were actually shorter in bipolar than in unipolar illness, this has not been an entirely consistent finding.

References: Perris (1966, 1982), Bebbington (1982).

5.38 **(a) F (b) T (c) T (d) T (e) F.**

"Secondary mania" refers to manic behaviour with or without grandiose delusions, and it can arise due to various organic illnesses. The drugs which cause it tend to be those that affect monoaminergic neurotransmitter function.

Reference: Cummings (1985).

5.39 (a) T (b) F (c) F (d) F (e) F.

(b) Puerperal psychosis is probably more common after Caesarian section, presumably due to the additional stress which this entails.

(c) There is usually a "lucid interval" of at least 2 days before the onset of psychiatric symptoms post-partum, and the commonest time for puerperal psychosis to be recognised is between 10 and 20 days after delivery.

(d) The majority of puerperal psychoses are depressive or manic illnesses.

(e) There is very often a good response to ECT, even although the symptomatology is not entirely typical of depressive psychosis.

References: Cox (1983), Kendell (1985).

5.40 (a) T (b) F (c) T (d) T (e) F.

(a), (c), (d) Emil Durkheim (1858-1917), a French sociologist, was particularly interested in the social factors relating to suicide. He introduced three categories of suicide. "Egoistic" suicide refers to a suicide precipitated by the individual losing his sense of belonging to the community such that he has to fall back on rules of conduct based on self interest. "Anomic" suicides are those which follow, for example, major social change or unrest such that there is a lack of "collective order". "Altruistic" suicides refer to those suicides committed for the good of society. The ritualized disembowelment ("hara-kiri") by the Japanese Samurai illustrates this category.

Reference: Gelder et al (1983).

5.41   (a) F (b) T (c) T (d) F (e) T.

(a), (b)   The loss of father at any time or the loss of mother after 11 years do not increase vulnerability.

(d)   Three or more children at home under the age of 14 years increase vulnerability.

Reference: Brown (1978).

5.42   (a) F (b) F (c) F (d) T (e) T.

(a)   In psychoanalytic theory, anxiety is distinguished from fear; the latter is a reaction to a real external danger, whereas anxiety occurs in response to internal, intrapsychic threat in the form of the threatened emergence of forbidden impulses.

(b)   Projection is the attribution of one's own unacceptable qualities or feelings to others. This underlies paranoid thinking. Displacement is the defence associated with phobias, whereby sexual anxiety is said to be transferred or displaced from its original source to an apparently innocuous object or situation.

(c)   Repression is an <u>unconscious</u> process whereby unacceptable impulses, ideas or memories are prevented from entering consciousness. Supression is a deliberate and <u>conscious</u> intention to avoid thinking about certain material.

5.43 (a) F (b) T (c) F (d) F (e) F.

(a) Although modelling may be effective for a few patients,
this is not generally the case. "Response prevention" is
a more effective behavioural approach.

(b) This is a major characteristic and distinguishes this
behaviour from other urges such as drinking and gambling.

(c), (d) The patient is always aware that they are his own
actions and not the product of external influences or of
hallucinations.

(e) It is common for children to develop rituals, such as
avoiding walking on the cracks in paving stones, but such
actions are not the same as obsessional rituals because
the children regard them as natural, and they do not find
them distressing. This cannot be said of patients who
develop obsessional rituals.

Reference: Freeman (1983a).

5.44 (a) F (b) T (c) F (d) T (e) F.

(a), (b), (d) Fenichel was the first to point out that our
fears are often disguised by certain attitudes and
behaviour which represent a denial that we are threatened.
The counterphobic individual may expose himself
persistently and deliberately to those circumstances he
actually fears. For example, in an attempt to master his
fear of heights the individual may become a mountaineer or
steeplejack.

(c) Countertransference is the term given to particular
responses of the therapist to the patient; these may be a
misrepresentation of reality due to the therapist's own
unresolved conflicts.

Reference: Fenichel (1934).

5.45 (a) T (b) T (c) F (d) T (e) T.

(a) This syndrome can give rise to a number of physical symptoms due to physiological changes induced by over-breathing. Consequently, it can mimic other conditions which may result in referral to a variety of specialties before it is diagnosed correctly.

(c) The peak age of occurrence is between 15 and 30 years.

(e) Air swallowing may give rise to epigastric distress and gastrointestinal symptoms.

Reference: Pincus (1978).

5.46 (a) F (b) T (c) F (d) F (e) T.

(a), (b) Bradycardia is usual. In association with cold extremities, hypotension and a generally hypodynamic circulation, this probably represents the body's physiological response to the low food intake : a form of "hibernation".

(c) Leukopenia is usual.

(d) Axillary and pubic hair is retained.

(e) The mechanism whereby ankle oedema arises is not fully understood, but is thought to be related to hypoproteinaemia and electrolyte imbalance.

References: Crisp (1980), Fairburn (1983a).

5.47 (a) F (b) F (c) T (d) T (e) F.

(a), (b) Bingeing, vomiting and purgative abuse have almost universally been found to indicate a poorer prognosis in anorexia nervosa.

References: Steinhausen and Glanville (1983), Vandereycken and Pierloot (1983).

5.48 **(a) T (b) F (c) F (d) F (e) F.**

(b)   The prevalence of obesity is highest in the lower
socioeconomic groups.

(d), (e)   It is now fairly well established that many obese
people eat no more than people of normal weight, and that
there is thus often a significant constitutional component
to the problem.

Reference: Fairburn (1983a).

5.49 **(a) T (b) F (c) T (d) F (e) T.**

Briquet's syndrome occurs almost exclusively in women and
has an onset in early adult life.   The patient presents
with a large number of different physical symptoms
relating to various organ systems, for which no organic
cause can be found.   Multiple operations and addiction to
prescribed drugs frequently occur.   Patients suffering
from this condition (also known as St Louis hysteria)
often exhibit prominent hysterical personality traits.
Psychiatric treatment is rarely successful, and indeed is
rarely acceptable to the patient, who retains "physical"
explanations for her symptoms.

Reference: Kendell (1983b).

5.50 (a) T (b) T (c) F (d) F (e) T.

(b) Nightmares are anxiety dreams, occurring in paradoxical
sleep, and should be distinguished from "night terrors"
which are transient experiences during orthodox sleep.

(c) Bruxism is of no psychiatric significance, although it can
be precipitated by psychotropic drugs.

(d) The EEG during sleep walking is not that of full
consciousness.

(e) Reduced and broken sleep is a feature of anorexia, and it
has been suggested that the weight loss in depressives may
be the cause of their early morning wakening.

Reference: Oswald (1983).

5.51 (a) F (b) F (c) F (d) F (e) F

(c) "Amentia" is a term used to describe an inborn mental
defect in contrast to an acquired dementia in later life.

(d) "Anhedonia" was first employed by Ribot, a French
psychologist, to refer to a chronic lack of pleasure. It
is a striking feature in psychotic depression when the
patient loses all pleasure from previously pleasurable
activities.

(e) "Anaclitic" defines relationships which are characterized
by emotional dependence on others.

5.52 (a) F (b) F (c) T (d) F (e) F

(a) There is no good evidence that women have increased rates of depressive psychosis in the perimenopausal years, or that "involutional melancholia" exists as a separate diagnostic entity.

(d), (e) When psychiatric symptoms do occur at the menopause they have been found not to be related temporally to "hot flushes", indicating that changes in oestrogen levels are unlikely to underlie such psychiatric symptoms. Oestrogen replacement therapy is thus not a rational treatment.

References: Ballinger (1978), Weissman (1979).

5.53 (a) T (b) T (c) F (d) F (e) F.

(c), (d) Compared to male homosexuals, lesbians are more likely to display a positive dislike of the opposite sex. They are more likely than males to be interested in cohabitation with a sexual partner and having a child either naturally or by adoption.

Reference: West (1983).

5.54 (a) F (b) T (c) F (d) T (e) T.

(a), (c) Insomnia and tachycardia occur.

Reference: Victor (1983).

5.55   (a) T (b) F (c) T (d) F (e) F.

(a), (c)   Since the 1950's, the cost of alcohol as a proportion
of average weekly income has fallen dramatically, while
alcohol consumption has risen steeply.   Kendell et al
(1983) showed that the 1981 budget, in which there was a
rise in the price of alcohol relative to income for the
first time in many years, caused a fall in alcohol
consumption in respondents interviewed before and after
the price increases.   This decrease in consumption
occurred even among the heavier "dependent" drinkers who
are sometimes thought to be immune to changes in price.

(b)   France leads the European "league table" with the highest
per capita alcohol consumption.

(e)   Overall per capita consumption is very similar in both
countries.   Scottish drinkers tend to drink in fewer
heavier sessions, thus probably accounting for their
increased rates of alcohol related disorders.

References: Kendell et al (1983), Ritson and Chick (1983).

5.56   (a) F (b) T (c) F (d) F (e) T.

(a), (c)   Cocaine is a powerful CNS stimulant, with similar
pharmacological properties to amphetamines.   It produces
increased energy, wakefulness, appetite suppression and
euphoria, as well as having peripheral sympathomimetic
effects.

(d)   As with amphetamines, true physical dependence probably
does not develop.

Reference: Ghodse (1983).

5.57 (a) F (b) T (c) T (d) T (e) F.

Under the Misuse of Drugs (Notification of and Supply to Addicts) Regulations 1973, if any doctor sees a patient whom he considers to be, or suspects of being, addicted to cocaine or any of the opiate drugs, then he is required to notify the Chief Medical Officer of the Home Office in writing within 7 days.

5.58 (a) F (b) T (c) T (d) F (e) F.

(a) Alcohol may provoke a latent predisposition to jealousy but it is rarely a primary cause of morbid jealousy.

(e) De Clèrambault's syndrome is also known as "psychose passionelle". This is a disorder in which a female has a delusional belief that a man, often older and of a higher social class than herself, is deeply in love with her.

Reference: Cobb (1979).

5.59 (a) T (b) T (c) T (d) F (e) T.

(d) The peak incidence is 45 years for women.

Reference: Scott (1978), Strachan (1981).

5.60 (a) T (b) T (c) T (d) T (e) T.

REFERENCES

ABRAMS, R. AND TAYLOR, M. A. (1981) "Importance of schizophrenic symptoms in the diagnosis of mania". American Journal of Psychiatry, 138, 658-661.

ALEXANDER, F. (1980) "Psychoanalytic therapy". In: Theories of Counselling and Psychotherapy, 3rd Edition, (Ed. C. H. Patterson). New York: Harper and Row.

AMBELAS, A. (1979) "Psychologically stressful events in the precipitation of manic episodes". British Journal of Psychiatry, 135, 15-21.

ANDERSON, J. (1982) "How to tackle multiple-choice question papers". Hospital Update, 8, 593-596.

AYLLON, T. AND AZRIN, N. H. (1968) The Token Economy: a Motivational System for Therapy and Rehabilitation. New York: Appleton-Century-Crofts.

BALLINGER, C. B. (1975) "Psychiatric morbidity and the menopause: screening of a general population sample". British Medical Journal, 3, 344-346.

BANCROFT, J. H. J. (1983) "Sexual disorders". In: Companion to Psychiatric Studies, 3rd Edition, (Eds. R. E. Kendell and A. K. Zealley). Edinburgh: Churchill Livingstone.

BANDURA, A. (1969) Principles of Behaviour Modification. New York: Holt, Rinehart and Winston.

BARNES, T. R. E. AND BRIDGES, P. K. (1982) "New generation of antidepressants". In: Drugs in Psychiatric Practice, (Ed. P.J. Tyrer). London: Butterworths.

BASS, C. (1984) "Type A behaviour: recent developments". Journal of Psychosomatic Research, 28, 371-378.

BEBBINGTON, P. E. (1982) "The course and prognosis of affective psychoses". In: Handbook of Psychiatry, Vol. 3, (Eds. J.K. Wing and L. Wing). Cambridge: Cambridge University Press.

BECK, A. T. (1976) Cognitive Therapy and the Emotional Disorders. New York: International Universities Press.

BERG, I. (1981) "Child psychiatry and enuresis". British Journal of Psychiatry, 139, 247-248.

BERG, I. (1983) "School non attendance". In: Handbook of Psychiatry, Vol. 4, (Eds. G. F. M. Russell and L. A. Hersov). Cambridge: Cambridge University Press.

BERGMANN, K. (1971) "The neuroses of old age" In: Recent Developments in Psychogeriatrics, (Eds. D. W. K. Kay and A. Walk). Kent: Headley Brothers.

BERGMANN, K. (1975) "The epidemiology of senile dementia". In: Contemporary Psychiatry, (Eds. T. Silverstone and B. Barraclough). Kent: Headley Brothers.

BERGMANN, K., FOSTER, E. M., JUSTICE, A. W. AND MATTHEWS V. (1978) "Management of the demented elderly patient in the community". British Journal of Psychiatry, 132, 441-449.

BERNE, E. (1961) Transactional Analysis in Psychotherapy. New York: Grove Press.

BERNE, E. (1964) Games People Play. New York: Grove Press.

BION, W. R. (1961) Experiences in Groups. London: Tavistock Publications.

BLUGLASS, R. (1979) "Incest". British Journal of Hospital Medicine, 22, 152-157.

BOND, M. R. (1979) Pain: its Nature, Analysis and Treatment. Edinburgh: Churchill Livingstone.

BOURNE, S. AND LEWIS, E. (1984) "Delayed psychological effects of perinatal deaths: the next pregnancy and the next generation". British Medical Journal, 289, 147-148.

BOYD, J. H. AND WEISSMAN, M. M. (1982) "Epidemiology". In: Handbook of Affective Disorders, (Ed. E. S. Paykel). Edinburgh: Churchill Livingstone.

BROWN, G. W. AND HARRIS, T. (1978) Social Orgins of Depression. London: Tavistock Publications.

BROWN, G. W., BIRLEY, J. L. T. AND WING, J. K. (1972) "Influence of family life on the course of schizophrenic disorders: a replication". British Journal of Psychiatry, 121, 241-258.

BROWN, G., CHADWICK, O., SHAFFER, D., RUTTER, M. AND TRAUB, M. (1981) "A prospective study of children with head injuries: (3) psychiatric sequelae". Psychological Medicine, 11, 63-78.

BURNS, T. AND CRISP, A. H. (1984) "Outcome of anorexia nervosa in males". British Journal of Psychiatry, 145, 319-325.

BYNUM, W. F. (1983) "Psychiatry in its historical context". In: Handbook of Psychiatry, Vol. 1, (Eds. M. Shepherd and O. L. Zangwill). Cambridge: Cambridge University Press.

CHADWICK, O., RUTTER, M., BROWN, G., SHAFFER, D. AND TRAUB, M. (1981) "A prospective study of children with severe head injuries: (2) cognitive sequelae". Psychological Medicine, 2, 49-61.

CHRISTIE, A. B. AND TRAIN, J. D. (1984) "Change in the pattern of care for the demented". British Journal of Psychiatry, 144, 9-15.

CHRISTIE-BROWN, J. R. W. (1983) "Paraphilias: sadomasochism, fetishism, transvestism and transsexuality". British Journal of Psychiatry, 143, 227-231.

CLARK, D. H. (1977) "The therapeutic community". British Journal of Psychiatry, 131, 553-564.

CLINICAL RESEARCH CENTRE, DIVISION OF PSYCHIATRY (1984) "The Northwich Park ECT trial: predictors of response to real and simulated ECT". British Journal of Psychiatry, 144, 227-237.

COBB, J. (1979) "Morbid jealousy". British Journal of Hospital Medicine, 21, 511-518.

COOPER, B. (1978) "Epidemiology". In: Schizophrenia: Towards a New Synthesis, (Ed. J. K. Wing). London: Academic Press.

COOPER, J. E. (1983) "Obsessional illness and personality". In: Handbook of Psychiatry, Vol. 4, (Eds. G. F. M. Russell and L. A. Hersov). Cambridge: Cambridge University Press.

COOPER, J. E. (1983) "Obsessional illness and personality". In: Handbook of Psychiatry, Vol. 4, (Eds. G. F. M. Russell and L. Hersov). Cambridge: Cambridge University Press.

COPPEN, A. AND METCALFE, M. (1965) "Effects of a depressive illness on MPI scores". British Journal of Psychiatry, 111, 236-239.

COPPEN, A., BISHOP, M., BEARD, R. J., BARNARD, G. J. R. AND COLLINS, W. P. (1981) "Hysterectomy, hormones and behaviour: a prospective study". Lancet, i, 126-128.

CORBETT, J. (1983) "Childhood origins of obsessional disorders, stereotyped behaviour, tics and Tourette's syndrome, and stuttering". In: Handbook of Psychiatry, Vol. 4, (Eds. G. F. M. Russell and L. A. Hersov). Cambridge: Cambridge University Press.

CORBETT, J. A. AND TURPIN, G. (1985) "Tics and Tourette's syndrome". In: Child and Adolescent Psychiatry, 2nd Edition, (Ed. M. Rutter and L. Hersov). Oxford: Blackwell.

COX, J. L. (1983) "Psychiatric disorders of childbirth". In: Companion to Psychiatric Studies, 3rd Edition, (Eds. R. E. Kendell and A. K. Zealley). Edinburgh: Churchill Livingstone.

CREED, F. (1981) "Life events and appendicectomy". Lancet, i, 1381-1385.

CRISP, A. H. (1980) Anorexia Nervosa: Let Me Be. London: Academic Press.

CROW, T. J. (1983) "Is schizophrenia an infectious disease?" Lancet, i, 173-175.

CUMMINGS, J. L. (1985) "Organic delusions: phenomenology, anatomical correlations and review". British Journal of Psychiatry, 146, 184-197.

CUTTING, J. (1982) "Neuropsychiatric complications of alcoholism". British Journal of Hospital Medicine, 27, 335-342.

DEL ZOMPO, M., BOCCHETTA, A., GOLDIN, L. R., AND CORSINI, G. U. (1984) "Linkage between X-chromosome markers and manic-depressive illness: two Sardinian pedigrees". Acta Psychiatrica Scandinavica, 70, 282-287.

DEWHURST, K. (1969) "The neurosyphilitic psychoses today: a survey of 91 cases". British Journal of Psychiatry, 115, 31-38.

EDWARDS, G. AND GROSS, M. M. (1976) "Alcohol dependence - provisional description of a clinical syndrome". British Medical Journal, i, 1058-1061.

ELLIS, P. AND MELLSOP, G. (1985) "De Clerambault's syndrome - a nosological entity?" British Journal of Psychiatry, 146, 90- 95.

ELWOOD, P. C., SHINTON, N. K., WILSON, C. I. D., SWEETNAM, P. AND FRAZER, A. C. (1971) "Haemoglobin, vitamin B12 and folate levels in the elderly". British Journal of Haematology, 21, 557-563.

ENOCH, M. D. AND TRETHOWAN, W. H. (1979) Uncommon Psychiatric Syndromes, 2nd Edition. Bristol: Wright and Sons Ltd.

FAIRBURN, C. G. (1983a) "Eating disorders". In: Companion to Psychiatric Studies, 3rd Edition, (Eds. R. E. Kendell and A. K. Zealley). Edinburgh: Churchill Livingstone.

FAIRBURN, C. G. (1983b) "Bulimia nervosa". British Journal of Hospital Medicine, 29, 539-542.

FENICHEL, O. (1934) Outline of Clinical Psychoanalysis. New York: Norton.

FENTON, G. W. (1972) "Epilepsy and automatism". British Journal of Hospital Medicine, 7, 57-64.

FICHTER, M. M., DOERR, P., PIRKE, K. M. AND LUND, R. (1982) "Behaviour, attitude, nutrition and endocrinology in anorexia nervosa". Acta Psychiatrica Scandinavica, 66, 429-444.

FISHER, C. (1984) "Psychiatric aspects of shoplifting". British Journal of Hospital Medicine, 31, 209-212.

FOLSTEIN, M. F. AND McHUGH, P. R. (1983) "The neuropsychiatry of some specific brain disorders". In: Handbook of Psychiatry, Vol. 2, (Ed. M. H. Lader). Cambridge: Cambridge University Press.

FORD, M. J., EASTWOOD, J. AND EASTWOOD, M. A. (1982) "The Irritable Bowel syndrome: soma and psyche". Psychological Medicine, 12, 705-707.

FRANKL, V. (1968) Psychotherapy and Existentialism. New York: Simon and Schuster.

FREEMAN, C. P. (1983) "Neurotic disorders". In: Companion to Psychiatric Studies, (Eds. R. E. Kendell and A. K. Zealley), 3rd Edition. Edinburgh: Churchill Livingstone.

FREEMAN, C. P. (1983a) "Neurotic disorders" In: Companion to Psychiatric Studies, 3rd Edition, (Eds. R. E. Kendell and A. K. Zealley). Edinburgh: Churchill Livingstone.

FREEMAN, C. P. (1983b) "Personality disorders". In: Companion to Psychiatric Studies, 3rd Edition, (Eds. R. E. Kendell and A. K. Zealley). Edinburgh: Churchill Livingstone.

FREEMAN, C. P. (1983c) "ECT and other physical therapies". In: Companion to Psychiatric Studies, 3rd Edition, (Eds. R. E. Kendell and A. K. Zealley). Edinburgh: Churchill Livingstone.

FREUD, A. (1936) The Ego and the Mechanisms of Defence. London: Hogarth Press.

GATH, A. (1985) "Chromosomal anomalies". In: Child and Adolescent Psychiatry, 2nd Edition, (Eds. M. Rutter and L. Hersov). Oxford: Blackwell.

GATH, D., COOPER, P. AND DAY, A. (1982a) "Hysterectomy and psychiatric disorder: (I) Levels of psychiatric morbidity before and after hysterectomy". British Journal of Psychiatry, 140, 335-342.

GATH, D., COOPER, P., BOND, A. AND EDWARDS, G. (1982b) "Hysterectomy and psychiatric disorder: (II) Demographic, psychiatric and physical factors in relation to psychiatric outcome". British Journal of Psychiatry, 140, 343-350.

GELDER, M. G. (1983) "Anxiety and phobic disorders, depersonalization and derealization". In: Handbook of Psychiatry, Vol. 4, (Eds. G. F. M. Russell and L. A. Hersov). Cambridge: Cambridge University Press.

GELDER, M., GATH, D. AND MAYOU, R. (1983) "Suicide and deliberate self-harm". Oxford Textbook of Psychiatry. Oxford: Oxford University Press.

GHODSE, A. H. (1983) "Drug dependence and intoxication". In: Handbook of Psychiatry, Vol. 2, (Ed. M. H. Lader). Cambridge: Cambridge University Press.

GIBBENS, T. C. N. AND ROBERTSON, G. (1983) "A survey of the criminal careers of hospital order patients". British Journal of Psychiatry, 143, 362-369.

GIBBONS, J. L. (1982) "Manic-depressive psychoses: mania". In: Handbook of Psychiatry, Vol. 3, (Eds. J. K. Wing and L. Wing). Cambridge: Cambridge University Press.

GIBSON, H. B. (1977) Hypnosis: its Nature and Therapeutic Uses. London: Owen.

GLICK, I. D. AND KESSLER, D. R. (1974) Marital and Family Therapy. New York: Grune and Stratton.

GOLD, P. W., KAYE, W., ROBERTSON, G. L., AND EBERT, M. (1983) "Abnormalities in plasma and CSF arginine vasopressin in patients with anorexia nervosa". New England Journal of Medicine, 308, 1117-1123.

GOLDBERG, D. (1983) "Depressive reactions in adults". In: Handbook of Psychiatry, Vol. 4, (Eds. G. F. M. Russell and L. A. Hersov). Cambridge: Cambridge University Press.

GRAHAM, P. AND RUTTER, M. (1985) "Adolescent disorders". In: Child and Adolescent Psychiatry, 2nd Edition, (Eds. M. Rutter and L. A. Hersov). Oxford: Blackwell.

GRAHAME, P. S. (1982) "Late paraphrenia". British Journal of Hospital Medicine, 27, 522-528.

GRAHAME, P. S. (1984) "Schizophrenia in old age (late paraphrenia)". British Journal of Psychiatry, 145, 493-495.

GURLAND, B., COPELAND, J., KURIANSKY, J., KELLEHER, M., SHARPE, L. AND DEAN, L. L. (1983) The Mind and Mood of Aging: Mental Health Problems of the Community Elderly in New York and London. New York: The Haworth Press.

GURMAN, A. S. AND KNISKERN, D. P. (1981) Handbook of Family
Therapy. New York: Brunner/Mazel.

HACHINSKY, V. C., ILIFF, L. D. AND ZILKHA, E. (1975) "Cerebral
blood flow in dementia". Archives of Neurology, 32,
632-637.

HAGNELL, O., LANKE, J., RORSMAN, B. AND OJESJO, L. (1982) "Are
we entering an age of melancholy?" Psychological Medicine,
12, 279-289.

HALL, E., SLIM, E., HAWKER, F. AND SALMOND, C. (1984) "Anorexia
nervosa: long-term outcome in 50 female patients". British
Journal of Psychiatry, 145, 407-413.

HAMILTON, M. (1985) Fish's Clinical Psychopathology. Bristol:
Wright.

HARDEN, R. McG., BROWN, R. A., BIRAN, L. A., DALLAS ROSS W. P.
AND WAKEFORD, R. E., (1976) "Multiple choice questions : to
guess or not to guess". Medical Education, 10, 27-32.

HARE, E. H. (1979) "Schizophrenia as an infectious disease".
British Journal of Psychiatry, 135, 468-473.

HERSOV, L. (1985a) "Emotional disorders". In: Child and
Adolescent Psychiatry, 2nd Edition, (Eds. M. Rutter and L.
Hersov). Oxford: Blackwell.

HERSOV, L. (1985b) "School refusal". In: Child and Adolescent
Psychiatry, 2nd Edition, (Eds. M. Rutter and L. Hersov).
Oxford: Blackwell.

HERSOV, L. (1985c) "Faecal soiling". In: Child and Adolescent
Psychiatry, 2nd Edition, (Ed. M Rutter and L. Hersov).
Oxford: Blackwell.

HOBBS, M. (1984) "Crisis intervention in theory and practice: a
selective review". British Journal of Medical Psychology,
57, 23-34.

HOLLAND, A. J., HALL, A., MURRAY, R., RUSSELL, G. F. M. AND
CRISP, A. H. (1984) "Anorexia nervosa: a study of 34 twin
pairs and one set of triplets". British Journal of
Psychiatry, 145, 414-419.

HSU, L. K. G. (1983) "The aetiology of anorexia nervosa".
Psychological Medicine, 13, 231-238.

HUDSON, J. I., POPE, H. G., JONES, J. M. AND YURGELUN-TODD, D. (1983) "Family history study of anorexia nervosa and bulimia". British Journal of Psychiatry, 142, 133-138.

IVERSEN, L. L. (1978) "Biochemical and pharmacological studies: the dopamine hypothesis". In: Schizophrenia: Towards a New Synthesis, (Ed. J. K. Wing). London: Academic Press.

JANOV, A. (1970) The Primal Scream. New York: Dell Publishing Company.

JARMAN, C. M. B. AND KELLETT, J. M. (1979) "Alcoholism in the general hospital". British Medical Journal, ii, 469-472.

JENNER, P. AND MARSDEN, C. D. (1982) "Antiparkinsonian and antidyskinetic drugs". In: Drugs in Psychiatric Practice, (Ed. P. J. Tyrer). London: Butterworths.

JOHNSON, D. A. W. (1981) "Studies of depressive symptoms in schizophrenia". British Journal of Psychiatry, 139, 89-101.

JOHNSTON, D. (1978) "Clinical applications of biofeedback". British Journal of Hospital Medicine, 20, 561-566.

JONES, M. (1976) The Maturation of the Therapeutic Community. New York: Human Sciences Press.

KAY, D. W. K. (1976) "The depressions and neuroses of later life". In: Recent Advances in Clinical Psychiatry, No. 2, (Ed. K. Granville-Grossman). Edinburgh: Churchill Livingstone.

KAY, D. W. K. (1978) "Assessment of familial risks in the functional psychoses and their application in genetic counselling". British Journal of Psychiatry, 133, 385-403.

KAYE, W. H., EBERT, M. H., RALEIGH, M. AND LAKE, C. R. (1984) "Abnormalities in CNS monoamine metabolism in anorexia nervosa". Archives of General Psychiatry, 41, 350-355.

KAZDIN, A. E. (1982) "History of behaviour modification". In: International Handbook of Behaviour Modification and Therapy, (Eds. A. S. Bellack, M. Hersen and A. E. Kazdin). New York: Plenum Press.

KENDELL, R. E. (1983a) "Schizophrenia". In: Companion to Psychiatric Studies, 3rd Edition, (Eds. R. E. Kendell and A. K. Zealley). Edinburgh: Churchill Livingstone.

KENDELL, R. E. (1983b) "Hysteria". In: Handbook of Psychiatry, Vol. 4, (Eds. G. F. M. Russell and L. A. Hersov). Cambridge: Cambridge University Press.

KENDELL, R. E. (1983c) "Other functional psychoses". In: Companion to Psychiatric Studies, 3rd Edition, (Eds. R. E. Kendell and A. K. Zealley). Edinburgh: Churchill Livingstone.

KENDELL, R. E. (1985) "Emotional and physical factors in the genesis of puerperal mental disorders". Journal of Psychosomatic Research, 29, 3-11.

KENDELL, R. E., DE ROUMANIE, M. AND RITSON, E. B. (1983) "Effect of economic changes on Scottish drinking habits, 1978-82". British Journal of Addiction, 78, 365-379.

KENDELL, R. E., RENNIE, D., CLARK, J. A. AND DEAN, C. (1981) "The social and obstetric correlates of psychiatric admission in the puerperium". Psychological Medicine, 11, 341-50.

KOGEORGOS, J. AND SCOTT, D. F. (1981) "Biofeedback and its clinical applications". British Journal of Hospital Medicine, 25, 601-605.

KOLVIN, I. (1983) "Speech and language disorders of childhood in children of average intelligence". In: Handbook of Psychiatry, Vol. 4, (Eds. G. F. M. Russell and L. A. Hersov). Cambridge: Cambridge University Press.

KRAUPL TAYLOR, F. (1983) "Descriptive and developmental phenomena". In: Handbook of Psychiatry, Vol. 1, (Eds. M. Shepherd and O. L. Zangwill). Cambridge: Cambridge University Press.

KREITMAN, N. (1983) "Suicide and parasuicide". In: Companion to Psychiatric Studies, 3rd Edition, (Eds. R. E. Kendell and A. K. Zealley). Edinburgh: Churchill Livingstone.

LEVY, R. AND POST, F. (1982) "The dementias of old age". In: The Psychiatry of Late Life, (Eds. R. Levy and F. Post). Oxford: Blackwell.

LISHMAN, W. A. (1973) "The psychiatric sequelae of head injury: a review". Psychological Medicine, 3, 304-318.

LISHMAN, W. A. (1978) Organic Psychiatry: The Psychological Consequences of Cerebral Disorder. Oxford: Blackwell.

LOUDON, J. B. (1983) "Drug treatments". In: Companion to Psychiatric Studies, 3rd Edition, (Eds. R. E. Kendell and A. K. Zealley). Edinburgh: Churchill Livingstone.

LUNZER, M. (1975) "Encephalopathy in liver disease". British Journal of Hospital Medicine, 13, 33-44.

MACKAY, A. V. P. (1982) "Antischizophrenic drugs". In: Drugs in Psychiatric Practice, (Ed. P. J. Tyrer). London: Butterworths.

MACRAE, A. K. M. (1983) "Forensic psychiatry". In: Companion to Psychiatric Studies, 3rd Edition, (Eds. R. E. Kendell and A. K. Zealley). Edinburgh: Churchill Livingstone.

MARKS, I. (1982) "Drugs combined with behavioural psychotherapy". In: International Handbook of Behaviour Modification and Therapy, (Eds. A. S. Bellack, M. Hersen, and A. E. Kazdin). New York: Plenum Press.

MARKS, I. M., STERN, R. S., MAWSON, D., COBB, J. AND McDONALD, R. (1980) "Clomipramine and exposure for obsessive-compulsive rituals". British Journal of Psychiatry, 136, 1-25.

MASTERS, W. H. AND JOHNSON, V. E. (1966) Human Sexual Response. Boston: Little, Brown and Company.

McCLURE, G. M. G. (1984) "Trends in suicide rate for England and Wales 1975-80". British Journal of Psychiatry, 144, 119-126.

MELLOR, C. S. (1970) "First-rank symptoms of schizophrenia". British Journal of Psychiatry, 117, 15-23.

MELLOR, C. S. (1975) "The epidemiology of alcoholism". In: Contemporary Psychiatry, (Eds. T. Silverstone and B. Barraclough). Kent: Headley Brothers.

MEZEY, G. C. (1985) "Rape: victiminological and psychiatric aspects". British Journal of Hospital Medicine, 33, 152-158.

MINDHAM, R. H. S. (1974) "Psychiatric aspects of Parkinson's disease". British Journal of Hospital Medicine, 11, 411-414.

MINDHAM, R. H. S. (1982) "Tricyclic antidepressants". In Drugs in Psychiatric Practice, (Ed. P. J. Tyrer). London: Butterworths.

MORAN, E. (1983) "Gambling". In: Handbook of Psychiatry, Vol. 4, (Eds. G. F. M. Russell and L. A. Hersov). Cambridge: Cambridge University Press.

MRAZEK, D. AND MRAZEK, P. (1985) "Child maltreatment". In: Child and Adolescent Psychiatry, 2nd Edition, (Eds. M. Rutter and L. Hersov). Oxford: Blackwell.

MURRAY, R. M. AND McGUFFIN, P. (1983) "Genetic aspects of mental disorders". In: Companion to Psychiatric Studies, 3rd Edition, (Eds. R. E. Kendell and A. K. Zealley). Edinburgh: Churchill Livingstone.

OKEN, D. (1985) "Gastrointestinal disorders". In: Modern Synopsis of Comprehensive Textbook of Psychiatry. (IV), (Eds. H. I. Kaplan and B. J. Sadock). Baltimore: Williams and Wilkins.

ORME, M. L. E. (1984) "Antidepressants and heart disease". British Medical Journal, 289, 1-2.

OSWALD, I. (1983) "Sleep disorders". In: Companion to Psychiatric Studies, 3rd Edition, (Eds. R. E. Kendell and A. K. Zealley). Edinburgh: Churchill Livingstone.

PARKES, C. M. (1985) "Bereavement". British Journal of Psychiatry, 146, 11-17.

PAYKEL E. S. (1982) "Medication and physical treatment of affective disorders". In: Handbook of Psychiatry, Vol. 3, (Eds. J. K. Wing and L. Wing). Cambridge: Cambridge University Press.

PAYKEL, E. S. (1978) "Contribution of life events to causation of psychiatric illness". Psychological Medicine, 8, 245-253.

PERRIS, C. (1966) "A study of bipolar (manic-depressive) and unipolar recurrent depressive psychoses". Acta Psychiatrica Scandinavica, Supplement 194.

PERRIS, C. (1982) "The distinction between bipolar and unipolar affective disorders". In: Handbook of Affective Disorders, (Ed. E. S. Paykel). Edinburgh: Churchill Livingstone.

PERRY, R. AND PERRY, E. (1982) "The ageing brain and its pathology". In: The Psychiatry of Late Life, (Eds. R. Levy and F. Post). Oxford: Blackwell.

PICKERING, G. (1979) "Against multiple choice questions". Medical Teacher, 1, 84-86.

PILOWSKY, I. (1983) "Hypochondriasis". In: Handbook of Psychiatry, Vol. 4, (Eds. G. F. M. Russell and L. A. Hersov). Cambridge: Cambridge University Press.

PINCUS, J. H. (1978) "Hyperventilation syndrome". British Journal of Hospital Medicine, 19, 312-313.

POPE, H. G., HUDSON, J. I., JONES, J. M. AND YURGELUN-TODD, D. (1983) "Bulimia treated with imipramine: a placebo controlled, double-blind study". American Journal of Psychiatry, 140, 554-558.

POST, F. (1982) "Functional disorders". In: The Psychiatry of Late Life, (Eds. R. Levy and F. Post). Oxford: Blackwell.

RABINS, P. V., MERCHANT, A. AND NESTADT, G. (1984) "Criteria for diagnosing reversible dementia caused by depression: validation by 2 year follow-up". British Journal of Psychiatry, 144, 488-492.

RACHMAN, S. J. (1982) "Obsessional compulsive disorders". In: International Handbook of Behaviour Modification and Therapy, (Eds. A. S. Bellack, M. Hersen and A. E. Kazdin). New York: Plenum Press.

REID, A. H. (1982) The Psychiatry of Mental Handicap. Edinburgh: Blackwell.

RICHMAN, N. (1985) "Disorders in pre-school children". In: Child and Adolescent Psychiatry, 2nd Edition, (Eds. M. Rutter and L. Hersov). Oxford: Blackwell.

RIMM, D. C. AND MASTERS, J. C. (1979) Behaviour Therapy, 2nd Edition. New York: Academic Press.

RIOCH, M. J. (1970) "The work of Wilfred Bion on groups". Psychiatry, 33, 56-66.

RITSON, E. B. AND CHICK, J. D. (1983) "Dependence on alcohol and other drugs". In: Companion to Psychiatric Studies, 3rd Edition, (Eds. R. E. Kendell and A. K. Zealley). Edinburgh: Churchill Livingstone.

ROBERTSON, E. E. AND KENNEDY, R. I. (1983) "Organic disorders". In: Companion to Psychiatric Studies, 3rd Edition, (Eds. R. E. Kendell and A. K. Zealley). Edinburgh: Churchill Livingstone.

ROGERS, C. R. (1951) Client-centered Therapy. Boston: Houghton Mifflin.

RUSSELL, G. F. M. (1970) "Anorexia nervosa: its identity as an illness and its treatment". In: Modern Trends in Psychological Medicine, 2, (Ed. J. H. Price). London: Butterworths.

RUSSELL, O. (1985) "Mental handicap". In: Current Reviews in Psychiatry, No. 1, (Eds. E.S. Paykel and H. G. Morgan). Edinburgh: Churchill Livingstone.

RUTTER, M. AND GOULD, M. (1985) "Classification". In: Child and Adolescent Psychiatry, 2nd Edition, (Eds. M. Rutter and L. Hersov). Oxford: Blackwell.

SANDERSON, P. H., (1973) "The 'don't know' option in MCQ examinations". British Journal of Medical Education, 7, 25-29.

SANDLER, J., DARE, C. AND HOLDER, A. (1970) "Basic psychoanalytic concepts: III Transference". British Journal of Psychiatry, 116, 667-672.

SELIGMAN, M. E. P. (1975) Helplessness. San Francisco: Freeman and Company.

SHAFFER, D. (1985) "Enuresis". In: Child and Adolescent Psychiatry, 2nd Edition, (Ed. M. Rutter and L. Hersov). Oxford: Blackwell.

SHIELDS, J. (1978) "Genetics". In: Schizophrenia: towards a new synthesis, (Ed. J. K. Wing). London: Academic Press.

SHULMAN, R. (1967) "Psychiatric aspects of pernicious anaemia: a prospective controlled investigation". British Medical Journal, iii, 266-270.

SNAITH, P. (1981) *Clinical Neurosis*. Oxford: Oxford University Press.

SOURINDRHIN, I. (1985) "Solvent misuse". *British Medical Journal*, 290, 94-95.

STAMPFL, T. G. AND LEVIS, D. J. (1967) "Essentials of implosive therapy: a learning - therapy - based psychodynamic behavioural therapy". *Journal of Abnormal Psychology*, 72, 496-503.

STEINHAUSEN, H. C. AND GLANVILLE, K. (1983) "Follow-up studies of anorexia nervosa: a review of research findings". *Psychological Medicine*, 13, 239-249.

STEPHENS, J. H., ASTRUP, C. AND MANGRUM, J. C. (1966) "Prognostic factors in recovered and deteriorated schizophrenics". *American Journal of Psychiatry*, 122, 1116-1121.

STORR, A. (1973) *Jung*. London: Fontana Modern Masters.

SURRIDGE, D. (1969) "An investigation into some psychiatric aspects of multiple sclerosis". *British Journal of Psychiatry*, 115, 749-764.

SYZMANSKI, L. S. AND CROCKER, A. C. (1985) "Mental retardation". In: *Modern Synopsis of Comprehensive Textbook of Psychiatry*, (IV), (Eds. H. I. Kaplan and B. J. Sadock). Baltimore: Williams and Wilkins.

TARSH, M. J. AND ROYSTON, C. (1985) "A follow-up study of accident neurosis". *British Journal of Psychiatry*, 146, 18-25.

TAYLOR, E. A. (1983) "Disturbances of toilet function". In: *Handbook of Psychiatry*, Vol. 4, (Eds. G. F. M. Russell and L. A. Hersov). Cambridge: Cambridge University Press.

THORLEY, A. P. (1982) "Alcohol". In: *Drugs in Psychiatric Practice*, (Ed. P. J. Tyrer). London: Butterworths.

TILLETT, R. (1984) "Gestalt therapy in theory and practice". *British Journal of Psychiatry*, 145, 231-235.

TREDGOLD, R. F. AND SODDY, K. (1970) *Mental Retardation*, 11th Edition. London: Baillière Tindall and Cassell.

TRIMBLE, M. R. (1981) _Neuropsychiatry_. Chichester: John Wiley and Sons.

TYRER, P. J. (1982a) "Anti-anxiety drugs". In: _Drugs in Psychiatric Practice_, (Ed. P. J. Tyrer). London: Butterworths.

TYRER, P. J. (1982b) "Monoamine oxidase inhibitors and amine precursors". In: _Drugs in Psychiatric Practice_, (Ed. P. J. Tyrer). London: Butterworths.

TYRER, S. AND SHAW, D. M. (1982) "Lithium carbonate". In: _Drugs in Psychiatric Practice_, (Ed. P. J. Tyrer). London: Butterworths.

TYRER, S. AND SHOPSIN, B. (1982) "Symptoms and assessment of mania". In: _Handbook of Affective Disorders_, (Ed. E. S. Paykel). Edinburgh: Churchill Livingstone.

VAILLANT, G. E. (1964) "Prospective prediction of schizophrenic remission". _Archives of General Psychiatry_, 11, 509-518.

VANDEREYCKEN, W. AND PIERLOOT, R. (1983) "The significance of subclassification in anorexia nervosa: a comparative study of clinical features in 141 patients". _Psychological Medicine_, 13, 543-549.

VAUGHN, C. E. AND LEFF, J. P. (1976) "The influence of family and social factors on the course of psychiatric illness: a comparison of schizophrenic and depressed neurotic patients". _British Journal of Psychiatry_, 129, 125-137.

VESSEY, M. P., McPHERSON, K., LAWLESS, M. AND YEATES, D. (1985) "Oral contraception and serious psychiatric illness: absence of an association". _British Journal of Psychiatry_, 146, 45-49.

VICTOR, M. (1983) "Mental disorders due to alcoholism". In: _Handbook of Psychiatry_, Vol 2, (Ed. M. H. Lader). Cambridge: Cambridge University Press.

WALKER, L. G. (1982) "The behavioural model". In: _Models for Psychotherapy: a Primer_. J. D. H. Haldane, D. A. Alexander and L. G. Walker. Aberdeen: Aberdeen University Press.

WALSH, B. T., STEWART, J. W., ROOSE, S. P., GLADIS, M. AND GLASSMAN, A. H. (1984) "Treatment of bulimia with phenelzine: a double-blind, placebo-controlled study". Archives of General Psychiatry, 41, 1105-1109.

WEIGHILL, V. E. (1983) "Compensation neurosis: a review of the literature". Journal of Psychosomatic Research, 27, 97-103.

WEINSTEIN, M. R. (1980) "Lithium treatment of women during pregnancy and in the post-delivery period". In: Handbook of Lithium Therapy, (Ed. F. N. Johnson). Lancaster: MTP Press.

WEISSMAN, M. M. (1979) "The myth of involutional melancholia". Journal of the American Medical Association, 242, 742-744.

WEST, D. J. (1983) "Homosexuality and lesbianism". British Journal of Psychiatry, 143, 221-226.

WEST, D. J. (1985) "Delinquency". In: Child and Adolescent Psychiatry, 2nd Edition, (Eds. M. Rutter and L. Hersov). Oxford: Blackwell.

WHITELY, J. S. (1970) "The psychopath and his treatment". British Journal of Hospital Medicine, 3, 263-270.

WILLI, J. AND GROSSMANN, S. (1983) "Epidemiology of anorexia nervosa in a defined region of Switzerland". American Journal of Psychiatry, 140, 564-567.

WILSON, G. T. (1980) "Behaviour modification and the treatment of obesity". In: Obesity, (Ed. A. J. Stunkard). Philadelphia; Saunders.

WING, J. K. (1982a) "Psychosocial factors influencing the onset and course of schizophrenia". In: Handbook of Psychiatry, Vol. 3, (Eds. J. K. and L. Wing). Cambridge: Cambridge University Press.

WING, J. K. (1982b) "Course and prognosis of schizophrenia". In: Handbook of Psychiatry, Vol. 3, (Eds. J. K. and L. Wing). Cambridge: Cambridge University Press.

WOLFF, S. (1983a) "Psychiatric disorders of childhood". In: Companion to Psychiatric Studies, 3rd Edition, (Eds. R. E. Kendell and A. K. Zealley). Edinburgh: Churchill Livingstone.

257

WOLFF, S. (1983b) "Childhood origins of hysterical personality disorder and of hysterical conversion syndromes: hysterical conversion symptoms in childhood". In: Handbook of Psychiatry, Vol. 4, (Eds. G. F. M. Russell and L. A. Hersov). Cambridge: Cambridge University Press.

WOLFF, S. (1983c) "Determinants of emotional and conduct disorders in childhood". In: Handbook of Psychiatry, Vol. 4, (Eds. G. F. M. Russell and L. A. Hersov). Cambridge: Cambridge University Press.

WOLFF, S. (1985) "Non-delinquent disturbances of conduct". In: Child and Adolescent Psychiatry, 2nd Edition, (Eds. M. Rutter and L. Hersov). Oxford: Blackwell.

YULE, W. AND RUTTER, M. (1985) "Reading and other learning difficulties". In: Child and Adolescent Psychiatry, 2nd Edition, (Eds. M. Rutter and L. Hersov). Oxford: Blackwell.

ZEALLEY, A. K. (1983) "Mental handicap". In: Companion to Psychiatric Studies, 3rd Edition, (Eds. R. E. Kendell and A. K. Zealley). Edinburgh: Churchill Livingstone.

ZILBOORG, G. (1967) A History of Medical Psychology. New York: Norton.

INDEX